Oxford Medical

Problem-solving treatment for anxiety and depression

Problem-solving treatment for anxiety and depression

a practical guide

Dr Laurence Mynors-Wallis
University of Southampton
Alderney Hospital, Poole, Dorset, UK

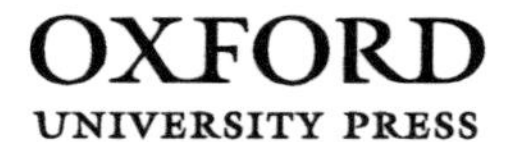

4-06

OXFORD
UNIVERSITY PRESS

Great Clarendon Street, Oxford OX2 6DP

Oxford University Press is a department of the University of Oxford.
It furthers the University's objective of excellence in research, scholarship,
and education by publishing worldwide in

Oxford New York

Auckland Cape Town Dar es Salaam Hong Kong Karachi
Kuala Lumpur Madrid Melbourne Mexico City Nairobi
New Delhi Shanghai Taipei Toronto

With offices in

Argentina Austria Brazil Chile Czech Republic France Greece
Guatemala Hungary Italy Japan Poland Portugal Singapore
South Korea Switzerland Thailand Turkey Ukraine Vietnam

Published in the United States
by Oxford University Press Inc., New York

First published 2005

British Library Cataloguing in Publication Data
Data available

Library of Congress Cataloging in Publication Data

Mynors-Wallis, Laurence.
Problem-solving treatment for anxiety and depression : a practical guide / Laurence
Mynors-Wallis.
Includes bibliographical references and index.
1. Problem-solving therapy. 2. Anxiety–Treatment. 3. Depression, Mental–Treatment.
[DNLM: 1. Mental Disorders–therapy. 2. Problem Solving. 3. Psychotherapy–
methods. WM 400 M997p 2005] I. Title.
RC489.P68M96 2005 616.89'14–dc22 2005015505

Typeset by Newgen Imaging Systems (P) Ltd., Chennai, India
Printed in Great Britain
on acid-free paper by
Biddles Ltd, King's Lynn

ISBN 0–19–852842–6 (Pbk.) 978–0–19–852842–5 (Pbk.)

10 9 8 7 6 5 4 3 2 1

For Rachel, Daniel, and Ben

Acknowledgements

Firstly I would like to pay tribute to my mother who instinctively taught me the importance of trying to sort out problems for myself and hence fostered independent thought, useful not only for problem-solving, but also for life. I have been fortunate in the many people who have helped me over the years that I have researched and taught problem-solving treatment. Dr Dennis Gath first introduced me to problem-solving and to the possibilities that the treatment offered for both research and practical application. He also taught me the importance of clear thinking and writing—skills very useful for problem-solving. Ann Day and Faith Barbour were stalwarts of support during my early problem-solving studies, working beyond what was necessary with commitment and good humour. Mark Hegel helped develop and improve upon the first problem-solving manual. Yo Davies has been an invaluable and much esteemed colleague with whom I have worked closely in developing problem-solving training. Evelyn van Weel–Baumgarten has, more recently, contributed further developments with training and has helped open up possibilities for the use of problem-solving in Europe. Julie Street, my personal assistant, has coped with the many changes to the manuscript in her unfailingly helpful and supportive way. Lastly, and most importantly, my wife Anne has provided me with the love and encouragement without which challenges such as this book could not be undertaken.

Contents

Chapter 1

Introduction to problem-solving treatment

Outline of problem-solving treatment

Problem-solving treatment is a brief, psychological treatment that has been adapted and developed for particular use in primary care. As the name suggests, the treatment takes a problem-solving approach to the management of psychological disorders. The theoretical assumption underpinning problem-solving is that psychological symptoms of depression and anxiety are often caused by practical problems people face in their everyday lives. Patients themselves readily recognize this link between their problems and the development of their illness. Problem-solving treatment, therefore, is often viewed by patients as a sensible and appropriate intervention.

Problem-solving treatment begins by establishing the link between the psychological symptoms that a patient is experiencing and the practical difficulties that they face. The treatment then offers a clear structure within which patients can resolve their problems, with the expectation that their symptoms will improve as their problems resolve. The treatment is very much a 'here and now' treatment, focusing on current difficulties that the patient is facing and setting goals for the future. The treatment does not dwell on past relationships and past mistakes.

There is both a behavioural and a cognitive aspect to problem-solving treatment. The behavioural component includes the setting of specific tasks designed to help the patient work through their problems. The cognitive component involves demonstrating to the patient that they need not be overwhelmed and beset by their problems, but rather there are practical and effective steps that they can take which will lead to problem resolution. Patients are thus helped to gain a sense of mastery over their difficulties.

Problem-solving treatment is collaborative, with the patient playing an active part in the recovery process. Problem-solving is also a relatively brief treatment and, because of this, there is little opportunity for patients to develop dependency on their therapist. An additional factor in avoiding dependency is that the treatment takes a skills-training approach. The patient is trained to use the problem-solving techniques to overcome their own problems. Following successful treatment with problem-solving, the patient does not feel that their improvement is due to a therapist, or a tablet, but rather that they have made themselves better by applying skills that they have learnt.

This book firstly sets out the evidence supporting the use of problem-solving treatment. The main focus is then to provide a detailed description of the problem-solving treatment process in sufficient depth so that would-be practitioners can use the techniques in their own practice.

The goals of problem-solving treatment

During problem-solving treatment, the therapist and patient attempt to achieve four major goals:

1. To increase the patient's understanding of the link between their current symptoms and their current everyday problems. Included in this goal is an understanding that problems are an expected part of everyday living, and that effective resolution of such problems will help to improve how the patient is feeling.
2. To increase the patient's ability to clearly define their current problems. In addition, the importance of setting concrete and realistic goals for problem-solving is stressed and practised.
3. To teach the patient a specific problem-solving procedure in an attempt to solve their problems in a structured way. Problem-solving skills are introduced and practised using the real-life problems the patient is currently attempting to solve.
4. To produce more positive experiences regarding the patient's ability to solve problems, thereby increasing their confidence in their problem-solving ability and their feelings of self-control

during problematic situations. After learning the techniques of problem-solving the patient should be better able to cope with problems in the future and thus avoid or minimize further emotional distress.

Why problem-solving treatment was developed

Problem-solving treatment was developed to meet the demand for a psychological treatment for common mental health disorders that is not only effective but also feasible. Effectiveness can be demonstrated by evaluating the treatment in randomized controlled trials. Feasibility refers to the need to have a psychological treatment that is readily available to patients who might benefit from it. In order for this to be the case, the treatment must be relatively brief, acceptable to patients, and, if possible, be delivered by non-mental health care specialists.

Psychological disorders are a major and growing cause of morbidity throughout the western world. These disorders include not only the so-called severe mental disorders such as schizophrenia and bipolar disorder, but also, and more commonly, neurotic disorders such as anxiety and depression. Information about the prevalence of these conditions was provided by the UK National Psychiatric Morbidity Survey (Jenkins *et al.* 1997) which sampled 13,000 adults aged 16–65 of whom 10,108 were successfully interviewed. This survey found that the overall one-week prevalence of neurotic disorders was 12.3% in males and 19.5% in females. These disorders are not only common but are also a cause of considerable morbidity. It has been estimated, for example, that depression is the fourth highest health cause of days lost from work, with the expectation that it will move to second place by the year 2020 (Murray and Lopez 1996).

In view of the frequency of psychological disorders in the general population, it is unsurprising that they are also common among people consulting their general practitioners. Various studies have used self-report questionnaires to screen for these disorders in primary care. These studies have found prevalence rates ranging from 16% to 43% of general practice attenders (Barrett *et al.* 1988). In the fourth National Morbidity Survey of England and Wales (McCormick *et al.* 1995), psychological disorders were found to be the third most common cause of consultation in primary care (the first two causes being disorders of the respiratory system and of the cardiovascular system).

In primary care, the common symptoms of psychological disorders were identified by Goldberg and Huxley (1992), who studied 88 people diagnosed as having a mental disorder in primary care. The most common symptoms were anxiety and worry (82 people), while despondency and sadness were also frequent (71 people). Other common symptoms were fatigue (71), sleep disturbance (50), and irritability (38). Psychological symptoms were often accompanied and masked by somatic (physical) symptoms. It is well recognized that in primary care many people with emotional disorders present with somatic rather than psychological symptoms.

It was originally thought that nearly all psychological disorders seen in primary care were transient responses to life's crises. It is now recognized, however, that not all of these conditions have a good prognosis. In a South London general practice, the outcome of psychological disorders over five years was determined from the practice records. It was found that a large proportion of these disorders ran a chronic or relapsing course. Thus, for patients given a new psychiatric diagnosis, 18% of the men and 35% of the women received a psychiatric diagnosis in each subsequent year (Cooper *et al.* 1969). In Warwickshire, Mann and colleagues (1981) carried out a one-year follow-up of 100 people diagnosed by their GP as having an emotional disorder (89 being diagnosed as having an anxiety or depressive disorder). The outcome for these people was not good. Although a quarter recovered in the first months of follow-up and did not relapse, about half had intermittent relapses, and a quarter had a chronic course with persisting symptoms and regular consultations. An 11-year follow-up was completed for this cohort (Lloyd *et al.* 1996) which found that about half had had a chronic course with either relapsing and remitting symptoms, or persistent symptoms. These patients not only had a high psychiatric morbidity but also had a high consultation rate for physical illness and an increased mortality from all causes.

Among patients seen in primary care, considerable social impairment can be caused by emotional disorders, particularly by depressive disorders. In a series of 207 attenders with depressive disorders, identified by GPs in six Manchester practices (Johnson and Mellor 1977), over half were unable to continue with their normal lives and had to make a major change in their lifestyle, such as discontinuing work. In the Medical Outcomes Study from the USA, patients with depression were compared with patients with any of eight chronic medical conditions (hypertension, diabetes, advanced heart disease, angina, arthritis, back problems, lung problems, and gastrointestinal disorders) (Wells *et al.* 1992). It was found that the patients with depression had significantly worse social functioning than did the patients with chronic medical conditions.

The financial cost of emotional disorders is considerable. An estimate was made of the economic cost of non-psychotic disorders seen in general practice in the UK in 1985 (Croft–Jeffreys and Wilkinson 1989). Direct treatment costs were £372 million; taking into account the lost productivity, however, the total cost was £5.6 billion. Although this is an old study, the message remains true: that the major cost of psychological disorders is not the cost of treatment but rather the social costs—in particular, days lost from work. In 2000, the total cost for adult depression in England was estimated at over £9 billion, of which £370 million were direct treatment costs; there were 110 million working days lost (Thomas and Morris 2003).

In summary, anxiety and depressive disorders are common; they are largely disorders of primary rather than secondary care. These disorders often run a chronic course, at considerable social and economic cost to the individual and the country.

Treatments for psychological disorders

Anxiety and depression are largely seen and treated in primary care settings without onward referral to specialist mental health services. It is estimated that less than one in ten patients with anxiety and depression are referred to specialist services. It is clearly the case, therefore, that any treatment for these disorders needs to be not only effective but also available and feasible within the primary care setting. Effective treatments for depression and anxiety include drug treatments, psychological treatments, and social interventions.

Drug treatments

There are many studies demonstrating the benefits of a variety of drug treatments for both depression and anxiety. Randomized controlled trials of antidepressant medication for both depressive and anxiety disorders show that between two thirds and three quarters of patients improve on medication over a six to twelve-week period. Unfortunately, recovery rates are only about 50% in real-life settings.

There are many reasons for the differences in outcome between the benefits from medication seen in clinical trials and the benefits in real-life settings. Firstly, many patients in clinical practice do not have the clearly defined, specific disorders of those patients recruited into clinical trials. It is probably the case, therefore, that for these more complex patients, outcomes are less good than for the trial patients. Another important factor is that patients seen in clinical trials are monitored much more closely than in clinical practice. Indeed, when patients are offered more assertive follow-up in clinical practice this can improve recovery rates. A third and important factor, however, limiting the value of antidepressant medication, is the fact that compliance with medication is often suboptimal, with over 50% of patients stopping their medication by four weeks. When questioned, patients give four main reasons for this:-

1. Troublesome side effects.
2. A belief that pills will not solve their problems.
3. A fear of dependence.
4. Not being aware of the length of time for which treatment should be continued.

Therefore, although medication is both convenient and effective for both depressive and anxiety disorders, there are significant limitations. If medication is to be used, doctors must offer clear and careful explanations setting out the potential benefits of treatment and allaying concerns.

Psychological treatments

There is a clear demand for increased availability of psychological treatments. A survey of public opinion conducted by the Royal College of General Practitioners and the Royal College of Psychiatrists found that 90% of the general public thought that depression should be treated with counselling, compared with only 24% who thought that treatment should involve antidepressants (Paykel *et al.* 1998).

As with medication, there are many studies demonstrating the value of psychological treatments for both depression and anxiety. The effective psychological treatments for both anxiety and depression are those time-limited, structured treatments, focusing more on the 'here and now', rather than on difficulties from the past. Scott (1998) identified the following common factors in effective psychological treatments:

1. The individual is provided with an understandable model of illness.
2. The therapy has a well planned rationale and is highly structured.
3. Plans for producing change are made in a logical sequence.
4. Therapy encourages use of skills to promote change.
5. Change is attributed to the individual's rather than therapist's skilfulness.
6. The individual develops a greater sense of self-efficacy.

Current psychological treatments of proven value for anxiety and depressive disorders include, in particular, cognitive behavioural and interpersonal therapies. These treatments depend on the availability of a suitably trained and experienced therapist and require therapy extending over several hours, typically 16–20. Patients often have a high regard for such treatments but, unfortunately, the lack of availability of suitable therapists means that, in many areas, such treatments are not available or there are lengthy waiting lists.

Social treatments

Social interventions for depression and anxiety (for example, providing meaningful daytime activities, befriending schemes, and providing practical help with childcare, housing, or debt) are also effective. These interventions make a lot of sense intuitively but have less of an evidence base supporting their use.

Problem-solving treatment

The development of problem-solving treatment has been informed by the need to develop a psychological treatment for anxiety and depressive disorders in primary care—that is, a brief but effective alternative to medication and the more lengthy specialist psychological treatments currently available.

Length of treatment

Problem-solving treatment is brief, typically lasting four to six sessions. The first two sessions are typically of an hour's duration; subsequent sessions are of 30 minutes' duration, although some patients and therapists may schedule longer appointments. Therefore, the entire treatment programme can be delivered in approximately three to four hours. The first three sessions are usually a week apart; subsequent sessions are spaced at longer intervals.

Who can benefit from treatment?

Problem-solving treatment has been demonstrated to be effective for the treatment of depression and other types of emotional distress, and to be effective for older adults as well as adults of working age. Therefore, many patients presenting to primary care can potentially benefit from the treatment. The 2004 National Institute for Clinical Excellence Guideline for the management of depression recommends the use of problem-solving therapy in both mild and moderate depression (NICE 2004). The evidence base for problem-solving treatment is set out in Chapter two.

Who can deliver the treatment?

Problem-solving treatment can be delivered by a variety of therapists, once they have been trained in the technique. The treatment has been shown to be effective when delivered by psychiatrists, family doctors, psychologists, and nurses. The treatment techniques are readily understood by practitioners experienced in other cognitive behavioural interventions. Practitioners used to delivering treatments of a more psychodynamic nature may need more training in order to ensure the problem-solving treatment remains focused and is delivered within the time-frames available in primary care.

Chapter 2

Evidence supporting the use of problem-solving treatment

Introduction

Problem-solving can be defined as the process by which an individual attempts to identify effective coping skills for specific problematic situations in everyday living. Problems are those situations for which an immediate and easily recognisable solution is not apparent. The impact of these problems upon an individual's psychological functioning depends on their particular circumstances. An individual's personal coping skills form a link between problems and whether psychological symptoms develop. These coping skills are the result not only of personality and previous experience, but also may fluctuate depending on whether the individual is suffering from a psychological illness. The appraisal of problems as challenging or threatening, and the individual's self-perception as possessing robust or fragile coping skills, will also play a part in whether problems lead to the development of psychological symptoms.

Negative life events are known to be linked to the aetiology of psychiatric disorders. New cases of neurotic disorder identified during one month by GPs in London were investigated by means of standardized clinical and social interviews. When compared with a matched control group of consulting patients, the index group was found to have experienced significantly more life events during the three months before the onset of illness. Events particularly associated with neurotic illness were unexpected crises and failure to achieve life goals. Whilst serious threatening events had an important aetiological role, minor events also played a contributory part (Cooper and Sylph 1973).

Life events and problems are not only clearly linked to the causation of psychological illness but also, weak problem-solving ability is linked to the aetiology and maintenance of psychological distress (Nezu *et al.* 1989). Related research has also addressed the influence of problem-solving coping as a buffering factor regarding the effects of negative life stress. For example, Billings and Moos (1981) found that individuals who engaged in more problem-focused coping responses in reaction to major negative life changes displayed fewer depressive symptoms.

The theoretical link between everyday problems, problem-solving skills, and psychological distress has led researchers on both sides of the Atlantic to develop and evaluate a cognitive behavioural treatment based on enhancing the patient's problem-solving skills. Research has evaluated problem-solving treatment in both group and individual forms for a range of psychiatric conditions including depression, emotional disorders, and following deliberate self-harm.

The most widely evaluated model of problem-solving treatment is based on the adaptation of problem-solving treatment for use in primary care by a research team in the United Kingdom (Mynors–Wallis 1996). This model of problem-solving has been particularly developed for application in busy and time-constrained primary care settings. It has also been developed so that non-mental health specialists in the primary care setting, such as nurses and interested physicians, can be trained to administer the treatment. This model of problem-solving treatment aims to enhance the patient's problem-solving skills over four to six treatment sessions. The evidence underpinning problem-solving treatment is set out in the following sections.

Major depressive disorders

As noted in Chapter one, there is a considerable demand for effective psychological treatments for depressive disorders as an alternative to antidepressant medication. Although antidepressant medication is both convenient and effective in the treatment of depression, there are significant disadvantages. Firstly, antidepressant drugs may have unpleasant side-effects. Secondly, patients have a fear of becoming dependent on medication. Thirdly, medication may seem irrelevant to many patients who feel beset with psychological and social problems. Indeed, there is good evidence that many depressive disorders are related to psychological and social problems. All these factors may result in poor compliance. These disadvantages highlight the need for a psychological treatment as an effective alternative to antidepressant drugs.

Several psychological treatments may be considered for the treatment of depressive disorders. The interventions for which there is best evidence are cognitive behaviour therapy and interpersonal psychotherapy. In cognitive therapy, the acute symptoms of depression are tackled through the use of behavioural and verbal techniques. Negative thoughts are identified and challenged in a collaborative, hypothesis-testing approach. Behavioural tasks are identified to check out the accuracy of negative beliefs. Later in treatment, interventions are targeted at challenging dysfunctional beliefs to try and reduce vulnerability to future episodes. In interpersonal psychotherapy, the underlying hypothesis and treatment rationale is that interpersonal problems are linked to depression. Therapy focuses on one or more of four areas of possible interpersonal difficulties—prolonged grief reactions, role disputes, role transitions, and interpersonal deficits. There is good evidence that both cognitive behaviour therapy and interpersonal therapy are effective interventions for depression, with equivalent efficacy to antidepressant medication (Geddes and Butler 2001).

Both cognitive behaviour therapy and interpersonal therapy have been evaluated for 12–16 treatment sessions, each lasting an hour. In many settings, there are neither sufficient therapists nor sufficient resources to provide such treatment. Problem-solving treatment delivered over fewer treatment sessions by less highly trained therapists has been evaluated as an alternative psychological treatment for depression.

The first problem-solving outcome study (Nezu 1986) for individuals with depression randomly assigned 26 depressed individuals to receive one of the following treatments:

1. Problem-solving treatment.
2. Problem-focused therapy.
3. Waiting list control.

The subjects were recruited from a newspaper advertisement and were all diagnosed as suffering from a unipolar depressive disorder according to research diagnostic guidelines.

Both active treatment programmes were delivered over eight, 90-minute sessions in group format. Problem-solving treatment included training in the areas of problem orientation, problem definition and formulation, generation of alternative solutions, decision making, solution implementation and verification. Individuals in the problem-focused therapy group received information that resolution of problematic situations and other sources of stress would lead to a decrease in depression but were not provided with a systematic model for problem resolution. They were encouraged to use the group sessions to discuss problems with other group members. Members of the waiting list control group were told that the programme was unable to accommodate any further members but, at the end of eight weeks, they could receive treatment if they still desired it. The results of this study, as determined by outcome on the Beck Depression Inventory (Beck *et al.* 1961)—a scale measuring depressive symptoms—are shown in Fig. 2.1 at two months' (post treatment) and at six months' follow-up for the three treatment groups.

On entry to the study, the three treatment groups did not differ significantly in mean scores on the Beck Depression Inventory. At the end of treatment, the problem-solving treatment group had lower depression scores than either of the other two groups. This difference was maintained at the six-month follow-up.

This study provided early evidence that the hypothesis linking problem-solving with symptom resolution was supported. However, treatment numbers were small. Participants were recruited via a newspaper advertisement rather than from patients seeking treatment from

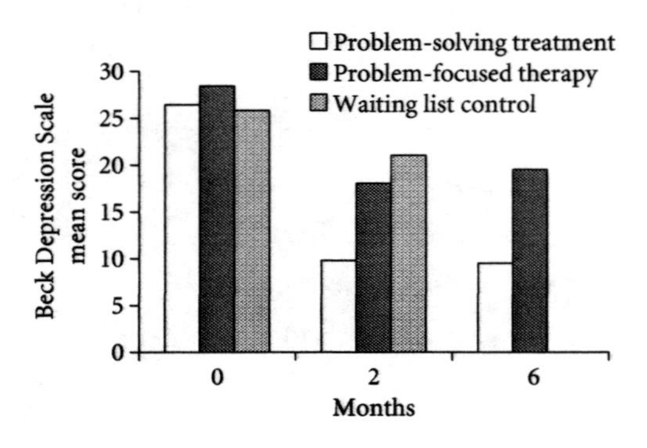

Fig. 2.1 Depressive symptoms at baseline and two months' and six months' follow-up for the three treatment groups.

their doctor. Also, the treatment was provided in a group format which, although cost effective in terms of time, is not liked by many patients.

Depressive disorders are, by and large, seen and treated in primary care without specialist referral. In the working conditions of primary care, time constraints and the restricted availability of trained psychologists limit access to psychological treatments. There were good reasons for evaluating the efficacy of problem-solving treatment for depressive disorders in primary care. Previous work using problem-solving treatment for patients following deliberate self-harm indicated that individual problem-solving treatment could be delivered in a brief, readily learnt format which was acceptable to patients (Hawton and Kirk 1989).

Against this background, a randomized controlled clinical trial was carried out to evaluate problem-solving treatment for major depression in primary care (Mynors–Wallis *et al.* 1995). The aim of this study was to answer two questions. In the treatment of major depression in primary care:

1. Is problem-solving treatment *effective*?
2. Is problem-solving treatment *feasible*?

The trial compared three treatments for major depression: problem-solving treatment; amitriptyline (an antidepressant) with standard clinical management; and drug placebo with standard clinical management. Each of the three treatments was given in six sessions over twelve weeks. The first session was scheduled to last 60 minutes, and the five subsequent sessions to last for 30 minutes each. The three treatments were given in primary care health centres or in patients' homes. The treatments were provided by three therapists, (one research psychiatrist and two research GPs). The therapists received systematic training in all three treatments.

The drug treatment was either amitriptyline or drug placebo. The administration of these substances was double-blind. All capsules were prescribed as for amitriptyline, the dose being increased to 150 mg over 10 days. In order to structure the drug treatment sessions, and to avoid the use of problem-solving techniques during these sessions, a manual was written for the drug treatments. This manual was based on one used in the NIMH Treatment of Depression

Collaborative Research Program (Fawcett *et al.* 1987). The therapist and patient spent the allocated time in discussing how the medication might be expected to work; what side-effects might be experienced; how these effects could be minimized; and how the patient's symptoms were progressing from session to session. Patients receiving the drug treatments were scheduled to receive the same amount of therapist time as those receiving problem-solving treatment.

Ninety-one patients entered the study. Assessments of the patients were carried out by independent research interviewers who were blind to the treatment given. These assessments were made at week 0 (pre-treatment), week 6 (halfway through treatment), and at week 12 (completion of treatment). The main outcome measures were the Hamilton Rating Scale for Depression (Hamilton 1967) and the Beck Depression Inventory (Beck *et al.* 1961).

This study provided evidence that problem-solving treatment is an effective treatment for depression. On entry to the study (week 0) the three treatment groups did not differ significantly in mean scores on the Hamilton Depression Scale. At week 6, the mean scores were problem-solving group 8.5; amitriptyline group 10.3, placebo group 13.8. At week 12, the mean scores were problem-solving group 7.1, amitriptyline group 8.1, placebo group 11.8. These results are shown graphically in Fig. 2.2.

Problem-solving treatment was statistically significantly more effective than placebo, but not significantly different from amitriptyline, at both six and twelve weeks.

It was of interest to know not only the mean overall outcome for the whole group of patients but also how many patients had fully

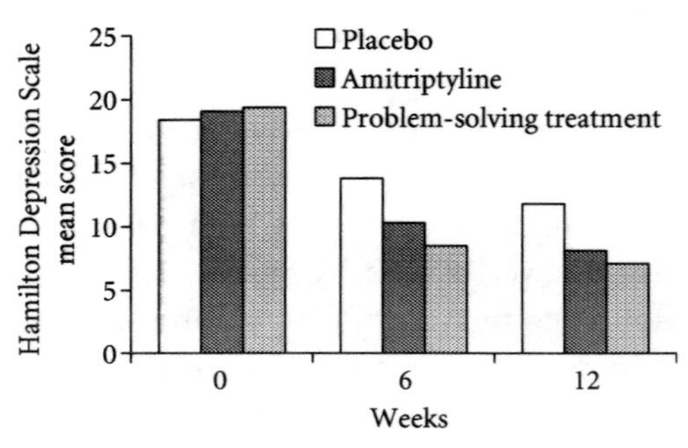

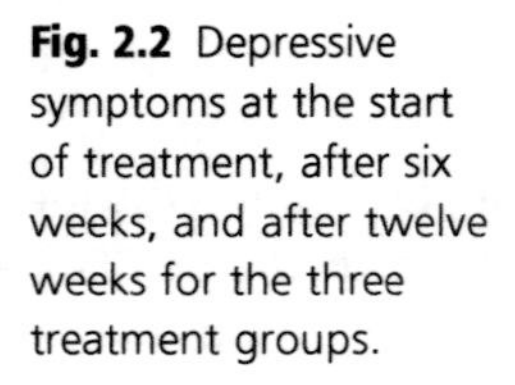
Fig. 2.2 Depressive symptoms at the start of treatment, after six weeks, and after twelve weeks for the three treatment groups.

recovered by the end of treatment. For this purpose, predetermined recovery criteria were used, as recommended by Frank *et al.* (1991). Thus, patients were categorized as recovered if they had end of treatment scores of 7 or less on the Hamilton Rating Scale. When this criterion was used, the proportions of patients who had recovered by week 12 were problem-solving 60%, amitriptyline 52%, placebo 27%.

This study showed that problem-solving was an effective treatment. The second important question was whether problem-solving treatment was feasible in primary care. To answer this, three issues were evaluated:

1. Was the duration of problem-solving treatment practicable?
2. Could members of a primary health care team deliver the treatment effectively?
3. Was the treatment acceptable to patients?

With regard to duration of treatment, for patients who completed all six treatment sessions, the mean overall therapy times were: problem solving, 3 h 24 min; amitriptyline, 3 h 3 min; placebo 2 h 55 min. In comparison with most other psychological treatments, the duration of problem-solving treatment was very brief.

The second issue was whether problem-solving treatment could be given by a primary care clinician rather than a mental health specialist. In this study, two GP therapists were used. For patients treated by the GPs, the outcome was as good as the outcome for patients treated by the psychiatrist. It is important to be cautious in interpreting this result because of the small number of therapists involved. The result, however, suggests that interested GPs can be trained to use problem-solving treatment effectively.

The final question was whether problem-solving treatment was acceptable to patients. The low drop-out rate (2 of 30 patients) suggested that patients found the treatment acceptable. This assumption was reinforced by the patients' answers to a self-report questionnaire. For example, among patients who completed treatment, the treatment was regarded as helpful by 100% of patients receiving problem-solving, compared with 83% receiving amitriptyline. When asked whether they were given help with problems, 96% of problem-solving patients answered positively, compared with 56% of amitriptyline patients.

Overall, the findings from this study indicated that problem-solving treatment was as effective as amitriptyline and more effective than drug placebo, was feasible in practice, and was well accepted by patients and family doctors.

A second study evaluating problem-solving treatment for major depression in primary care (Mynors–Wallis *et al.* 2000) was designed to answer two further questions. Firstly, is the combination of problem-solving treatment and antidepressant medication more effective than either treatment alone? Secondly, can the problem-solving treatment be delivered as effectively by suitably trained nurses as by GPs? In order to answer this question, four treatments for major depression in primary care were compared in a randomized controlled trial:

1. Paroxetine (an antidepressant) alone, given by research GPs.
2. Problem-solving treatment alone, given by research GPs.
3. Problem-solving treatment alone, given by research community nurses.
4. A combination of problem-solving treatment given by research community nurses and paroxetine given by research GPs.

Three research GPs and two research nurses from primary care were the therapists in the study. None had previous mental health experience outside primary care. All were trained in problem-solving treatment before the study commenced. Paroxetine was chosen as the comparator antidepressant because, at the time, it was a widely used antidepressant in primary care.

One hundred and fifty-one patients were enrolled in this study. Both the problem-solving and drug treatments were given in six sessions over a twelve-week period. The results of this study, as measured by the Hamilton Rating Scale for Depression at baseline and at 6, 12, and 52-week follow-up for all four groups, are shown in Fig. 2.3.

There was no significant difference between the four groups at baseline. There were no significant differences between the four groups at 6, 12, or 52-week follow-up on any of the outcome measures used.

There are four key messages from this study:

1. Further evidence that problem-solving treatment is an effective treatment for depressive disorders in primary care.

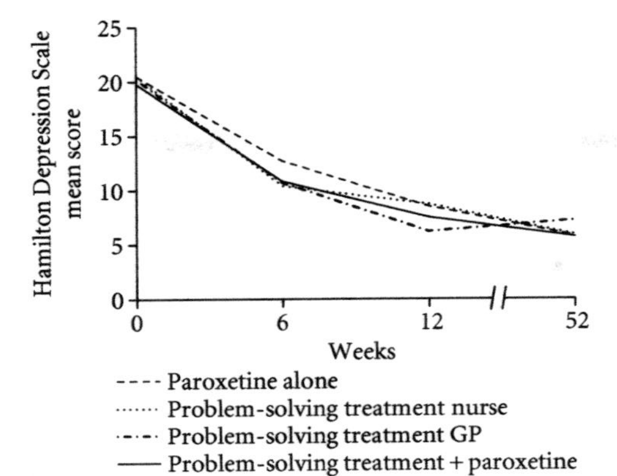

Fig. 2.3 Depressive symptoms at the start of treatment, at six weeks, at 12 weeks, and at 52-week follow-up for the four treatment groups.

2. Problem-solving treatment can be delivered by suitably trained nurses as effectively as by GPs.
3. The combination of problem-solving treatment and antidepressant medication is no more effective than either treatment alone.
4. Problem-solving treatment is likely to benefit patients who have a depressive disorder of moderate severity and who wish to participate in an active psychological treatment.

The next randomized controlled trial to evaluate problem-solving treatment for depressive disorders was a multicentre European study (Dowrick *et al.* 2000). This study set out to determine the acceptability of two psychological interventions for depressed adults in the community: problem-solving treatment and group psychoeducation. The study was set in nine urban and rural communities in Finland, Ireland, Norway, Spain, and the United Kingdom. Four hundred and fifty-two participants aged 18 to 65, identified through a community survey as having depressive or adjustment disorders, were randomly allocated to receive one of three interventions:

- Six individual sessions of problem-solving treatment (n = 128).
- Eight group sessions of a prevention depression course (n = 108).
- Waiting list control (n = 189).

The problem-solving treatment was as that described in the studies of Mynors–Wallis *et al.* (1995, 2000). The prevention of depression course was based on group psychoeducation, emphasising instruction rather than therapy and promoting relaxation, positive thinking, pleasant activities, and social skills. 63% of participants assigned to individual problem-solving treatment and 44% assigned to prevention of depression course completed the intervention. The proportion of each of the three groups recovered at six or twelve months was:

	At six months	At twelve months
Problem-solving treatment	59%	62%
Group psychoeducation	55%	53%
Waiting list	42%	61%

The proportion of participants who received problem-solving that were still depressive at six months was 17% less than for controls, giving a number needed to treat of six. There were also significant improvements in quality of life measures between those who had received problem-solving and the control group. The study concluded that, when offered to adults with depressed disorders in the community:

- Problem-solving treatment was more acceptable than a prevention of depression course.
- There was a significant improvement in the proportion of subjects who recovered from depression and in depression severity scores following problem-solving treatment compared with waiting list control.
- Problem-solving treatment improved quality of life.

Minor depression and dysthymia

Major depression describes depressive disorders in which patients experience not only low mood but also four or more of the key symptoms of depression (sleep disturbance, appetite disturbance, poor concentration, guilt, suicidal thoughts, anhedonia, psychomotor retardation, and fatigue) and have, in addition, a degree of social impairment. Patients who do not meet these diagnostic criteria, usually because of the presence of too few depressive symptoms, may nonetheless experience significant social impairment. The two depressive diagnoses which can be used to categorize such patients are minor depression and dysthymia. Minor depression describes the presence of low mood plus two more depressive symptoms.

Dysthymia describes low mood plus two depressive symptoms for a continuing period of two or more years. Both these disorders are common in primary care and, hence, there is a need to evaluate potentially effective and feasible treatments.

Problem-solving treatment was compared with paroxetine for the treatment of patients with minor depression or dysthymia in two communities in the United States (Lebanon, New Hampshire and Seattle, Washington) (Barrett *et al.* 2001). Two hundred and forty-one primary care patients (aged 18–59) with minor depression (n = 114) or dysthymia (n = 127) were randomized to receive paroxetine (10–40 mg per day), placebo, or individual problem-solving treatment. Of these, 191 patients (79%) completed all treatment visits. Depressive symptoms were measured using the 20-item Hopkins Depression Scale (Liepman *et al.* 1979) (HSCL-D-20). Remission was defined on the Hamilton Depression Rating Scale (Hamilton 1967) as less than or equal to 6 at 11 weeks.

All treatment conditions showed a significant decline in depressive symptoms over the 11-week study period. For patients with dysthymia, the remission rates for paroxetine (80%) and problem-solving treatment (57%) were significantly higher than for placebo (44%), with paroxetine being the more effective treatment. For patients with minor depression, the overall remission rate was 64% and similar for each treatment group (paroxetine 61%, problem-solving treatment 66%, placebo 66%). The conclusions from this study were that for patients with dysthymia, drug treatment should be the first-line treatment, but problem-solving treatment should be considered as a alternative treatment to medication. For patients with minor depression, watchful waiting, with regular face-to-face contact, should be the initial treatment of choice, with medication or problem-solving being used for those patients with persistent symptoms or increasing severity of symptoms over time.

In a study with a similar design to that just described, but an older cohort of patients, 415 primary care patients with minor depression (n = 204) or dysthymia (n = 211) were recruited from four US settings (Williams *et al.* 2000). Again, patients were randomly allocated to receive paroxetine (n = 137) 10–40 mg per day, placebo (n = 140), or individual problem-solving treatment (n = 138). All three groups received six visits over eleven weeks. The conclusions from this study were that paroxetine showed moderate benefit for depressive symptoms and mental health functioning in elderly patients with dysthymia and the more severely impaired elderly patients with minor depression. The benefits of problem-solving treatment were smaller and were more subject to site differences than those of paroxetine. One of the findings from this study was that therapist skill in problem-solving led to significantly greater benefits for the problem-solving treatment.

Quality improvement programmes for depression

Although there are effective psychological and pharmacological treatments for depression, poor compliance and lack of assertive follow-up for patients not responding to the initial treatment has meant that outcomes for patients in naturalistic settings are significantly less than the predicted outcomes derived from carefully controlled scientific studies. The failure to effectively implement evidence-based treatments has led to quality improvement programmes in primary care which have focused on ensuring that patients receive appropriate treatment until recovery (Katon *et al.* 1995, 1996, 1999).

The largest quality improvement programme for patients with depressive disorders has been undertaken in the United States (Unutzer 2001). This study enrolled 1801 patients from primary care, aged 60 years or over, with major depression, dysthymia, or both. The quality improvement programme focused on improving both the use of medication and psychological treatments. Problem-solving treatment was chosen as the psychological treatment in the programme. Patients were randomly allocated to either a collaborative care management programme (n = 906) or usual care (n = 895). Intervention patients had access for up to twelve months with a depression care manager, supervised by a psychiatrist and a primary care expert. The depression care manager offered education, support of antidepressant management, or problem-solving treatment. Patients had a choice at each stage of a stepped care programme of either medication or problem-solving treatment. The results at twelve months showed that 45% of the intervention patients had a 50% or greater reduction in depressive symptoms from baseline, compared with 19% of usual care participants. Intervention patients also experienced greater rates of depression treatment, more satisfaction with depression care, and greater quality of life.

The importance of this study is that it shows that problem-solving treatment can be integrated within a primary care setting alongside medication. Patients then have the option of either a psychological intervention for depression and/or a drug treatment. The possibility of such a choice of treatments, together with assertive case management, leads to significantly better outcomes than usual care.

Depression in older adults

In a US study, 75 older adults diagnosed with a major depressive disorder were randomly allocated to either problem-solving therapy or reminiscence therapy or waiting list control (Arean 1993). Problem-solving in this study was provided in the form of 20 weekly sessions of group treatment, as was the reminiscence therapy. At post-treatment, both the problem-solving treatment and reminiscence therapy conditions produced significant reductions in depressive symptoms compared with the waiting list control group. However, the problem-solving participants experienced significantly less depression than reminiscence therapy subjects. A significantly greater proportion of participants in problem-solving treatment, compared with reminiscence therapy, were rated as improved or in remission at post-treatment and follow-up.

In a small American study, 25 elderly patients with major depression and impairment in executive function were randomly allocated to receive problem-solving treatment or supportive therapy. Problem-solving treatment was more effective than supportive therapy in leading to remission of depression, fewer post-treatment depressive symptoms, and less disability. A substantial part of the change in depression and disability was explained by the subjects' improvement in problem-solving skills and in decision making (Alexopolous *et al.* 2003). One conclusion from this study was that problem-solving treatment may be an important therapeutic alternative to medication for patients with major depression and executive dysfunction who may otherwise remain symptomatic and disabled.

Depression and problem-solving treatment: conclusions

The studies reviewed demonstrate that problem-solving treatment has been evaluated in the treatment of depressive disorders for both adults and older people in Europe and the United States. The evidence suggests that problem-solving treatment:

- Is an effective treatment for major depression in primary care.
- Is more effective than placebo and as effective as antidepressant medication.
- Is an effective treatment when part of a stepped care quality improvement treatment programme.

There is less evidence that problem-solving is an effective treatment for minor depression and dysthymia. Problem-solving treatment should be considered as a second-line intervention for patients with minor depression who have not responded to watchful waiting and for patients with dysthymia who have failed to respond to antidepressant medication.

Problem-solving treatment has not yet been compared with other proven psychological treatments for depression, in particular cognitive behaviour therapy and interpersonal psychotherapy. Problem-solving treatment should not be considered as more effective than such interventions. The importance of problem-solving is that it is a brief and feasible psychological treatment which can be made widely available to patients as an effective alternative to medication.

Emotional disorders

Emotional disorders describe a range of disorders including adjustment disorders, anxiety disorders, mixed anxiety and depressive disorders, and minor depressive disorders. In primary care it can often be difficult to distinguish between such disorders using the psychiatric classifications used in secondary care. Patients commonly present with a mixture of anxious and depressive symptoms, often occurring in response to situational crises. Problem-solving treatment was considered a suitable therapy for such patients not least because these disorders often occur seemingly in response to life's difficulties.

The first controlled evaluation of problem-solving treatment for patients with emotional disorders was a result of findings in a study from Oxfordshire. This study had shown that for patients with a recent onset emotional disorder (predominantly anxiety), brief counselling by the GP, in the form of explanation, reassurance, and advice, was as effective as anxiolytic medication (Catalan *et al.* 1984). With either treatment about 60% of patients improved substantially within four weeks of the initial consultation, and a further 10% improved within six months. However, there remained 30% of patients with a poor prognosis, who were still significantly unwell six months after their initial consultation. The aim of the first study of problem-solving treatment in primary care was to discover whether problem-solving treatment would be effective for this group of patients.

One challenge when evaluating treatments for emotional disorders is that a significant proportion of patients improve with time and only minimal intervention. Hence, the first difficulty was to identify the poor prognosis patients from those who would improve with only minimal intervention. Poor prognosis was defined as patients remaining psychiatrically unwell six months after the initial consultation. There were no simple clinical or demographic variables that predicted, at the initial consultation, which patients would remain unwell six months later. However, the poor prognosis patients could be reliably identified four weeks after the initial consultation by a total score of 12 or above on the Present State Examination (PSE) (Wing *et al.* 1974)—a standardized psychiatric interview. Those patients with a score below 12 at the four-week assessment had only a 10% risk of being a 'case' on the PSE at six months, whereas a total score of 12 or above indicated a 66% risk.

For the study (Catalan *et al.* 1991), GPs referred patients, aged 18 to 65, who had recent onset complaints of anxiety, tension, depressed mood, irritability, sleep disturbance, or somatic symptoms not apparently due to physical illness. Four weeks later, a member of the research team visited the patient at home, took a history, and administered the PSE. Patients were selected for the study if their total score was 12 or more on the PSE and were then allocated randomly to problem-solving treatment or a control treatment. The control treatment was any treatment the GP chose to give, whether pharmacological, psychological, or social.

In this study, 113 potentially suitable patients were referred by GPs, 66 of whom had a PSE total score under 12 at four weeks and 47 had a PSE total score of 12 or more. These 47 patients with high scores at four weeks were randomly allocated to problem-solving treatment (21 patients) or to GP's usual treatment (26 patients). The problem-solving treatment consisted of four treatment sessions over six weeks given by a research psychiatrist.

Before treatment, the two patient groups were found to be well matched on PSE total scores (problem-solving group 16.6, control group 17.7). After eight weeks, both treatment groups had improved significantly, but the reduction in scores was significantly greater for the problem-solving group than for the control group (mean difference 3.7). At the final assessment (28 weeks), the problem-solving group showed further slight improvement, but this improvement was not significant compared to the post-treatment findings. At 28 weeks, the reduction in PSE total score since the start of treatment was significantly greater in the problem-solving group than the control group. Thus, treatment effects were maintained at follow-up. Figure 2.4 illustrates the results.

At the end of treatment, patients were given a checklist with which to identify elements of the treatment that they found helpful. Compared with control patients, significantly more problem-solving patients endorsed as helpful elements of problem-solving treatment such as problems were pinpointed, problems were broken into steps, help was given in deciding what to do, advice was given on tackling problems, plans were made as to what to do between meetings.

The conclusion from this study was that problem-solving treatment, given by a psychiatrist, was a feasible and effective treatment for emotional disorders of poor prognosis in primary care. It was liked by

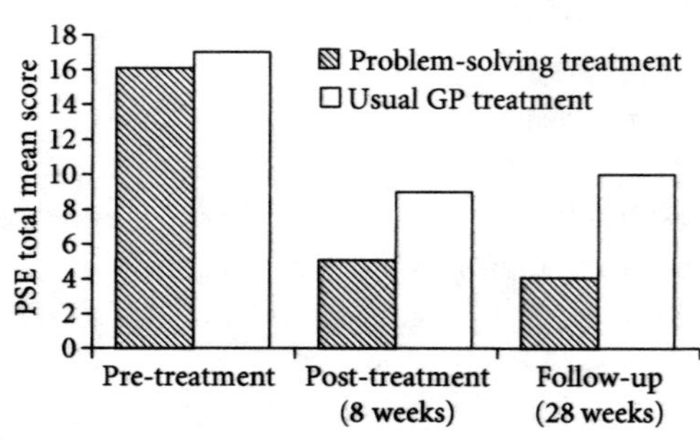

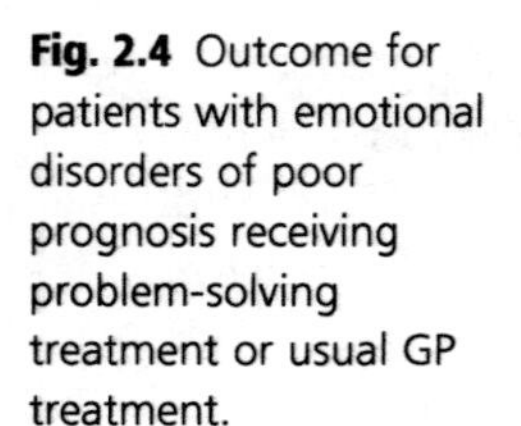

Fig. 2.4 Outcome for patients with emotional disorders of poor prognosis receiving problem-solving treatment or usual GP treatment.

patients (no drop-outs), and problem-solving techniques were identified as being helpful in recovery.

A second study evaluating problem-solving treatment in primary care for emotional disorders sought to evaluate the treatment as given by community nurses (Mynors–Wallis *et al.* 1997). Although interested GPs can be trained to use problem-solving techniques, it is difficult for them to find the time to provide this treatment for all their patients in need. Problem-solving treatment could be made more widely available if non-medical members of the primary care team (for example, community nurses) could be trained to use the technique effectively.

There is evidence that nurses can be trained to provide psychological treatments successfully. For example, in primary care, nurses have used behavioural methods to treat obsessional and phobic patients (Ginsberg *et al.* 1984). Nurses have also been used in primary care to try to improve compliance with antidepressant medication (Wilkinson *et al.* 1993). In hospitals, nurses have been trained to include problem-solving techniques in the counselling of patients after deliberate self-harm (Hawton and Kirk 1989; Salkovskis *et al.* 1990).

Six nurses were recruited for the study. They were nurses working in primary care without any specific psychiatric skills. Their training programme comprised two parts. The first part consisted of four half-day workshops led by a research psychiatrist and a clinical nurse specialist in behavioural psychotherapy. The workshops involved detailed theoretical training in problem-solving treatment and practical skill learning based on role play. The training techniques used are described in detail in Chapter 9. In the second part of the training programme, the nurses treated patients under close supervision. GPs were asked to refer patients for the training whom they thought might benefit from problem-solving treatment. Each patient was offered four to six sessions of problem-solving treatment. Videotaped recordings were made of each treatment session, and these were then used in supervision sessions to give the nurses detailed feedback about their problem-solving skills.

The results from the training phase of this study indicated that nurses could be trained in the use of problem-solving treatment techniques. Before and after ratings of the nurses' skills showed that, over the course of training, skills in problem-solving increased for all the nurses to above a predetermined satisfactory threshold level. It is important to note that the nurses required the practical hands-on experience of treating patients under supervision to bring about a satisfactory level of skill, and not simply attendance at the training workshops.

Once the nurses had completed the training phase of the study, their skills in problem-solving treatment were evaluated in a randomized controlled clinical trial. Patients with emotional disorders were referred by their GPs. These patients were allocated randomly to receive either problem-solving treatment given by a trained nurse therapist or usual GP treatment.

GPs were asked to identify patients aged 18 to 65 with emotional disorders of at least one month's duration. The GP reassessed the patient after four weeks, and then referred those patients with persistent symptoms into the study. This delay before referral into the study was an attempt to select out those patients with a good prognosis who would improve over the first four weeks irrespective of treatment received. The GP was asked to avoid starting psychotropic medication during the four-week waiting period. Referred patients were assessed, using standardized interview and self-report measures, on three occasions: before treatment, at the end of treatment (8 weeks), and at 26 weeks' follow-up.

There was no significant difference in the Present State Examination (PSE) (Wing *et al.* 1994) mean total scores between the two groups before treatment (problem-solving 13.2, treatment as usual 11.9). Outcome at 8 and 26 weeks showed little difference between the two groups on mean PSE scores: at 8 weeks (problem-solving 5.6, treatment as usual 8.1) or at 26 weeks (problem-solving 5.6, treatment as usual 5.6). The results on the other outcome rating scales used gave similar findings, with no differences in outcome between the problem-solving and control groups at either 8- or 26-week follow-up.

For patients allocated to problem-solving treatment, the median number of treatment sessions was four. The average number of consultations with a GP for problem-solving patients was 2.1 over the eight-week treatment phase. Among patients who received treatment as usual, the average number of consultations with the GP was 2.2 during the eight weeks after initial assessment.

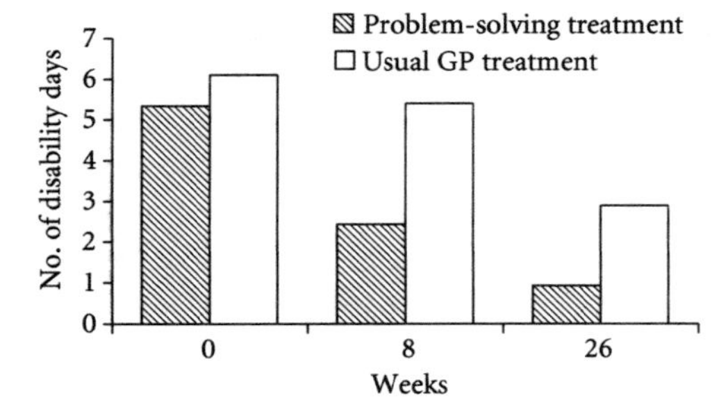

Fig. 2.5 Number of disability days in preceding month comparing outcome for problem-solving treatment and usual GP treatment.

There was a difference in outcome between the two groups in the number of disability days. Disability days are days on which the subject is unable to continue with their usual activities. At the pre-treatment assessment, the average number of disability days in the preceding month was 5.3 in the problem-solving group and 6.1 in the treatment as usual group. At the 8-week assessment, the corresponding numbers were 2.4 in the problem-solving group and 5.4 in the treatment as usual group ($p = 0.07$); at the 26-week assessment, the numbers were 0.9 in the problem-solving group and 2.9 in the treatment as usual group. These results are shown graphically in Fig. 2.5.

For patients in paid employment ($n = 42$), the total number of days off work sick over the six- month study period was 16.2 in the treatment as usual group and 4.3 in the problem-solving group, a mean difference of 11.9 days ($p = 0.05$). Thus, there is some evidence that problem-solving treatment reduced sickness-related days off work in comparison with treatment as usual.

The conclusions from this study were:

- Nurses can be trained in problem-solving techniques.
- Patients did not show any clinical benefit in terms of symptom reduction from the problem-solving treatment over and above the GP's usual treatment.
- There were considerable economic benefits from using the problem-solving treatment in terms of reduced disability days and reduced absenteeism.

It was surprising that the problem-solving treatment did not benefit the patients in this study over and above usual GP treatment.

This may be because the study design differed from the previous study of emotional problems of poor prognosis in primary care in that there was not a strict severity entry criteria for the study. Patients simply had to wait one month after initial assessment by the GP and then could be referred. In the event, there were almost no patients who were not entered into the study following their initial assessment. Patients in this study were not as unwell as patients in the previous study. A review of the diagnoses of study subjects were: mild depression 17%, moderate depression 40%, severe depression 9%, generalized anxiety disorder 3%, mixed anxiety and depression 11%, no psychiatric diagnosis 20%. Approximately half the patients, therefore, had an illness severity below that of a moderate depressive disorder. This study highlights the importance of selecting patients for treatment who have an illness severity which is likely to benefit from the intervention, over and above the passage of time and usual GP treatment.

A third study looking at problem-solving treatment for emotional disorders in primary care used community psychiatric nurses as problem-solving therapists (Simons *et al.* 2001). The study was designed to see whether patients with common emotional disorders could be helped by referral to specialist psychiatric nurses, compared with usual treatment from their GP. At present, in the UK, most specialist psychiatric nurses treat patients with severe mental illness such as schizophrenia and bipolar disorder. There is, however, pressure from GPs for more help in looking after patients with common mental disorders. As noted in Chapter one, these disorders are not only common but also are a cause of significant morbidity.

The trial design compared three treatments. In one of the treatment arms, patients were seen and treated by community psychiatric nurses using their experience and whatever skills they had, with the nurses deciding appropriate treatment (generic community psychiatric nurse care). In the second arm, the community psychiatric nurses were trained to deliver problem-solving treatment. In the third arm, patients received usual care from their GP.

The nurse therapists were recruited from two Mental Health Trusts in Southern England and represented a significant proportion of community psychiatric nurses working within those two organizations. These nurses were randomly allocated either to receive training in problem-solving treatment (as set out in Chapter 9) or to deliver generic community psychiatric nurse care. Patients were referred from the general practices serving the two Trusts. After the nurses delivering problem-solving treatment had been appropriately trained, 241 patients diagnosed by their GP as having depression, anxiety, or life difficulties were randomly allocated to receive one of three treatments:

1. Problem-solving treatment given by trained community psychiatric nurses.
2. Generic care given by community psychiatric nurses.
3. Usual care given by GPs.

The results from this study indicated that at 8- and 26-week follow-up, there was no difference in treatment outcome between the three treatment groups, either in terms of symptom severity or in terms of cost and days lost from work. The one significant difference between the groups was that patients who had received treatment from the community psychiatric nurses were much more satisfied with treatment received (85%) compared with patients who had received treatment from their GP alone (40%). This increased satisfaction was not linked to increased clinical improvement which showed no difference between the groups, but probably reflects softer and unmeasured factors.

A qualitative analysis was undertaken in which patients from all three treatment groups were interviewed. This analysis found that patients valued the opportunity to talk and be listened to, and appreciated that a genuine interest had been taken in them by the treating nurse, whether or not the nurse gave generic care or problem-solving treatment. This confirms the importance of the non-specific factors in psychological treatments and, in particular, the value of the patient–therapist relationship.

Emotional disorders and problem-solving treatment: conclusions

The three studies of emotional disorders in primary care described above recruited a broad group of patients, some of whom had chronic symptoms causing significant social impairment, but many of whom had relatively brief disorders which were not of great severity. Problem-solving treatment was shown to be effective when patients were carefully selected with clear threshold severity. The treatment has not been shown to be effective over and above usual GP treatment when such a threshold is not applied. This suggests, therefore, that problem-solving treatment for patients with emotional disorders should be reserved for those who have not improved with usual GP treatment. Such a conclusion would be in line with the conclusions from the studies of minor depression.

Deliberate self-harm

Many patients who harm themselves do so in the context of psychosocial stresses. These patients may or may not have diagnosable psychiatric disorders. They do, however, have problems which commonly include interpersonal difficulties (especially with partners and family members), unemployment, financial and housing problems, and social isolation. There is also evidence to suggest that many deliberate self-harm patients have specific deficits in their ability to solve the problems they face (Linehan *et al.* 1987; Schotte and Clum 1987). Therefore, therapeutic interventions based on problem-solving are regarded as a pragmatic approach for helping many people with suicidal behaviour (Hawton and Catalan 1987). Intuitively, problem-solving treatment would seem to be an appropriate and valid treatment for patients following deliberate self-harm.

Six studies have evaluated problem-solving treatment for patients following an episode of deliberate self-harm. In three of the trials (Patsiokas and Clum 1985; Hawton *et al.* 1987; Salkovskis *et al.* 1990), the descriptions of problem-solving treatment were very similar to the problem-solving methods used in the studies described for depression and emotional disorders. In Gibbons *et al.* (1978), the treatment (task-centred casework) focused on working on a single key problem. In McLeavey *et al.* (1994), particular attention was paid to improving problem-solving skills in general, as well as tackling current problems. Evans *et al.* (1999) provided a self-help manual for patients and included basic cognitive techniques to manage emotions and negative thinking, in addition to problem-solving.

The results from these trials were summarized and subjected to a meta-analysis (Townsend *et al.* 2001). The details of the separate trials, as summarized in the Townsend paper, are shown in Table 2.1.

The results of the meta-analysis can be considered under three headings:

1. Depression outcome

Those patients who had been offered problem-solving treatment had significantly greater improvement in scores for depression (standardized mean difference = −0.36; 95% confidence intervals −0.61 to −0.11). This difference means that patients who received problem-solving treatment had depression scores at the end of treatment an average of a third of a standard deviation lower than control patients.

2. Hopelessness

There was a significantly lower mean hopelessness score for patients who received problem-solving treatment compared with patients who received control treatment.

3. Improvement in problems

Significantly more patients who had received problem-solving treatment reported improvement in their problems (odds ratio = 2.31; 95% confidence interval 1.29 to 4.13) than patients who were in the control treatment group.

The authors conclude that problem-solving therapy for deliberate self-harm patients appears to produce better results than control treatment with regard to improvement in depression, hopelessness, and problems (Townsend *et al.* 2001). It remains uncertain whether these benefits lead to a reduction in self-harming attempts.

Problem-solving techniques are widely used when supporting patients following episodes of deliberate self-harm. Further research is needed to clarify its efficacy.

Table 2.1 Characteristics of the deliberate self-harm trials (Townsend *et al.* 2001)

Characteristics of participants				**Characteristics of interventions**	
	Numbers				
	E	**C**	**Repetition (%)**	**Experimental**	**Control**
Gibbons *et al.* 1978	200	200	Repeaters were included but proportion not significant	Crisis-orientated, time-limited task-centred social work at home. Problem-solving intervention that lasted for 3 months. Mean no. of sessions 9. Therapists = 2 social workers.	Routine treatment (referral back to GP, psychiatric referral, other referral)
Patsiokas & Clum 1985	5	5	Not significant	Interpersonal problem-solving skills training (D'Zurilla & Godfried 1971). Ten 1-hour sessions conducted over a 3-week period. Therapist = 1 clinical psychologist.	Individual therapy with clinical psychologist (content not specified)
Hawton *et al.* 1987	41	39	31	Outpatient problem-orientated therapy. Up to eight 1-hour sessions over an 8-week period. Therapists = 5 nurse counsellors.	GP care (e.g. individual support, marital therapy)
Salkovskis *et al.* 1990	12	8	100	Cognitive behavioural problem-solving treatment at home. Five 1-hour sessions over a month. Therapist = 1 community psychiatric nurse.	Treatment as usual (not described)
McLeavey *et al.* 1994	19	20	35–6	Interpersonal problem-solving skills training (D'Zurilla & Godfried 1971). Five 1-hour sessions at weekly intervals. Mean no. of sessions 5.3. Therapists = clinical psychologists and registrars in psychiatry.	Brief problem-solving therapy regarded as standard aftercare. Mean no. of sessions 4.2.
Evans *et al.* 1999	18	16	100	Manual assisted cognitive behavioural therapy for individuals with personality disorders) plus standard treatment. Treatment lasted 2–6 sessions. Time period for treatment not stated. Therapists = 1 psychiatrist, 2 nurses, 2 social workers.	Standard psychiatric treatment (e.g. psychiatrist, community mental health team, specialist social worker)

E = experimental group; C = control group

Other conditions in which problem-solving treatment has been evaluated

Psychological problems and diabetes

A time-limited, structured, problem-orientated intervention which aimed to decrease the severity of psychological problems and improve metabolic control in Type 1 diabetic patients with vascular complications has been evaluated (Didjurgeit *et al.* 2002). At six months, patients who had received problem-solving had a decreased severity of psychological problems and improved metabolic control of their diabetes.

Obesity

In a trial of 80 obese women who had completed 20 weekly group sessions of behaviour therapy, patients randomly allocated to problem-solving treatment had significantly greater long-term weight reductions than patients who had no further treatment. A larger percentage of problem-solving therapy patients achieved clinically significant losses of 10% more in body weight than did those patients who had no further contact (Perri *et al.* 2001).

Cancer support

A study of 341 first-degree relatives of women diagnosed with breast cancer randomly allocated them to problem-solving or a general counselling control group. The two groups did not differ at baseline or at follow-up in both cancer-specific and general distress. However, when problem-solving participants were divided into those who regularly practised the problem-solving treatment techniques and those who did not, a significant difference emerged. Participants who regularly practised the problem-solving techniques had significantly greater decreases in cancer-specific distress compared to the control group (Schwartz *et al.* 1998).

Palliative care

Emotional symptoms of depression and anxiety are common among palliative care patients. A small pilot study evaluated the feasibility and acceptability of using problem-solving treatment to treat these syndromes in patients receiving palliative care. There were significant difficulties in recruiting patients from palliative care for the study. However, many patients who had the problem-solving intervention described it as helpful in clarifying family and social issues (Wood and Mynors–Wallis 1997).

Supporting carers

Falloon *et al.* (1984) have described the use of problem-solving techniques within the context of family therapy for patients with schizophrenia. Problem-solving is used to clarify the particular problems each family faces and to enhance family coping skills. A problem-solving approach is also proposed for the carers of patients with physical needs (Houts *et al.* 1996). The intervention is designed to empower family members and patients for coping with illness and alleviating care giver stress.

Does problem-solving work by solving problems?

One of the problem-solving studies sought to answer the question whether problem-solving treatment works by resolving problems. In the study comparing problem-solving treatment, antidepressant medication, and the combination of the two treatments (Mynors–Wallis *et al.* 2000), possible mechanisms of action of the problem-solving intervention were evaluated. Two hypotheses were tested by comparison with drug treatment. Firstly, did problem-solving treatment work by achieving problem resolution? Secondly, did problem-solving treatment work by increasing the patients' sense of mastery and self-control (Mynors–Wallis 2002)?

In addition to rating clinical symptoms, patients were asked to rate the severity of their problems at baseline and at weeks 6 and 12. Patients identified up to three individual problems which were rated using the Personal Questionnaire Rapid Scaling Technique (PQRST) (Mulhall 1976). The PQRST involves the patient being asked to specify a problem (e.g. my husband does not help enough with the children). The interviewer then records the patient's responses to a series of paired adjectives asking how much of a problem something is. This process results in a rating of problem severity on a 10-point scale. In this way a standardized scoring system is used for individualized patient problems.

Self-control and sense of mastery were rated by patients on two 9-point anchored Likert scales, at baseline and at weeks 6 and 12. The two scales were:

1. I feel I have my life under control (self-control).
2. I feel overwhelmed by events (mastery).

Problem resolution

The graphs in Figs. 2.6 and 2.7 are the mean ratings of the severity of the patients' two main identified problems on the PQRST at baseline, at week 6, and at week 12. Results are shown according to treatment group.

These results do not suggest that problem-solving treatment brings about problem resolution more quickly than medication.

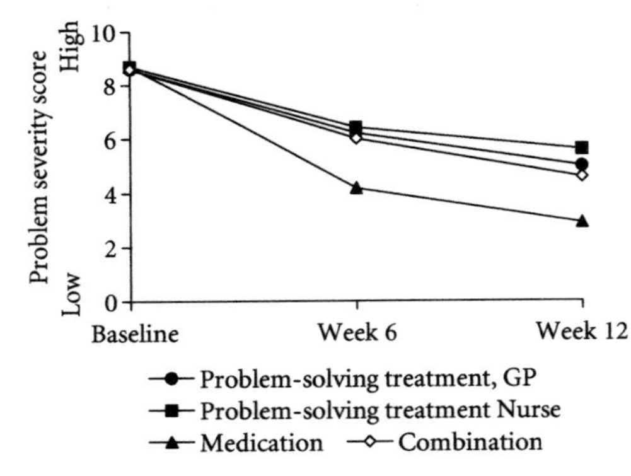

Fig. 2.6 Main problem identified: severity at baseline, at week 6 and at week 12, for the four treatment groups.

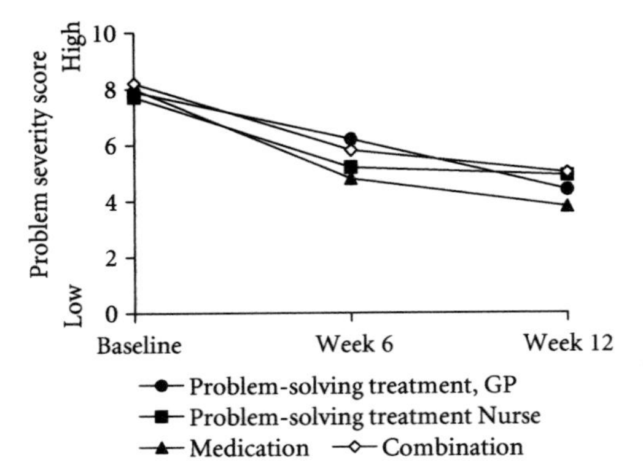

Fig. 2.7 Second problem identified: severity at baseline, at week 6 and at week 12, for the four treatment groups.

Self-control and mastery

The results from the self-control and mastery scales are given in Table 2.2 which reports firstly the number of patients who agreed or strongly agreed that their life was under control at each assessment point and, secondly, the number of patients who disagreed or strongly disagreed that they felt overwhelmed by events at each assessment point. The larger the number, the more patients who reported self-control and mastery.

These results do not show significant differences between patients who received problem-solving treatment and those who received medication to support the hypothesis that problem-solving enhances self-control or mastery as measured by the chosen scales. There were positive correlates between the severity of depressive symptoms and both problem severity scores and self-control and mastery scores.

Table 2.2 Results from self-control and mastery scales

Number of patients who agree or strongly agree with the statement 'I feel I have my life under control'			
	Baseline	**Week 6**	**Week 12**
PST, GP (n = 39)	2	3	13
PST, nurse (n = 41)	3	9	10
Medication (n = 36)	3	8	10
Combination (n = 35)	1	8	10
Number of patients who disagree or strongly disagree with the statement 'I feel overwhelmed by events'			
	Baseline	**Week 6**	**Week 12**
PST, GP (n = 39)	1	2	13
PST, nurse (n = 41)	4	5	8
Medication (n = 36)	2	9	11
Combination (n = 35)	5	9	13

PST = problem-solving treatment

The results from these analyses did not support the hypothesis that problem-solving treatment works through problem resolution or via self-control/mastery. A valid criticism, however, is that the study did not include an objective measure of problem severity. An outside view of the severity of the problem might have resulted in a different result. Also, in retrospect it might have been helpful to attempt to categorize the problems pre-treatment. Firstly, into problems likely to be soluble (in which case problem-solving might well have had a more clear mediating role). Secondly, problems could be categorized as likely to be insoluble (in which case problem-solving might have simply added to a sense of hopelessness—with the learning of coping skills likely to be more important). Thirdly, problems could be categorized as not problems at all but better understood as due to the patients' negative cognitions (and for these patients medication might well be most appropriate). This would be a fruitful area for further research.

Another point to consider is that perception of problem severity, self-control, and mastery may simply be proxy measures of depressed mood. A strong correlation was found between the self-control and mastery measures and the severity of symptoms on the Beck Depression Inventory. As patients' mood improved, so their concern about problems decreased. Similarly, as patients' mood improved, their sense of self-control and mastery increased. Simons *et al.* (1984), looking for differential effects of cognitive therapy versus nortriptyline pharmacotherapy on cognitive measures, reported a similar finding. They found that cognitive change occurred as much in pharmacotherapy as in cognitive therapy and concluded that cognitive measures behaved more as symptoms of depression rather than as causes. De Rubeis *et al.* (1990) considered this issue in relation to another study of cognitive therapy and pharmacotherapy and noted that depressive symptoms and the mechanisms of effective treatments are 'intertwined or reciprocally caused'. Similarly, Fava *et al.* (1994) found dysfunctional attitudes (a cognitive measure) to be positively associated with depression severity scores. They concluded that dysfunctional attitudes are a state-dependent symptom. It is probably the case that the measures chosen to determine the mechanism of problem-solving are similarly state-dependent symptoms rather than independent, mediating variables.

These findings from problem-solving treatment are thus in line with findings from cognitive therapy that the suggested mediators of the mechanism of action of the therapy cannot be proven. This may be because the proposed mediators are simply wrong or it may be that the proposed mediators are too closely linked with depressive severity to act as independent variables.

A final consideration is that if the measures chosen are not mediators for the mechanism of problem-solving treatment, what other mechanisms could be considered? One mechanism may simply be that of activity. Problem-solving treatment has a strong behavioural component with an emphasis on getting the patient to do activities. It may be that increased activity is the therapeutic mechanism. This is another area for research.

Chapter 3

The seven stages of problem-solving treatment

Introduction

Problem-solving treatment is a structured and focused treatment. There is an emphasis on getting the patient to quickly engage in activities which will bring about some early successes with the difficulties that they face. The challenge for the therapist is to facilitate the necessary patient activity and sense of achievement, without the patient feeling rushed and pushed into tasks for which they do not feel committed or adequately prepared. When patients, who have been treated with problem-solving, are asked what was helpful about the treatment, they identify not only the fact that they were helped to solve problems in a clear and structured way, but also that the therapist listened to their difficulties and helped to order their thoughts appropriately. The structure and focus of problem-solving treatment, therefore, must take place within a therapeutic context in which the patient feels supported and able to explain their thoughts and feelings.

Problem-solving treatment shares certain key characteristics with other cognitive behavioural treatments:

- The treatment focuses on the here and now rather than dwelling on issues from the past.
- The treatment has a clear rationale, structure, and organization.
- The direction of the treatment is provided by the therapist but the patient is encouraged to identify options and make decisions about which options to choose.
- The treatment provides techniques and skills which the patient practises outside treatment sessions.
- The treatment is time-limited with a clear number of treatment sessions being agreed with the patient at the start of treatment.

Problem-solving treatment is delivered over approximately six sessions. The content of each session will change, but elements of the structure of problem-solving should be identifiable in all. In the early sessions, more time will be spent by the therapist explaining how problem-solving treatment works, using examples from the patient's experience to bring this to life. In the later sessions, the patient and therapist should be able to use the problem-solving techniques without as much explanation.

The structure of problem-solving treatment can be considered to be a series of seven stages. This structure is an important component of the treatment. It is important for the therapist in that it enables treatment sessions to be focused on the key issues within the time available. It is important for the patient in that they learn a clear and structured approach to the management of problems which can clarify and order often vague and overwhelming problems. One of the skills of problem-solving is the ability to place patient's problems within the structure of the seven stages of treatment without the treatment appearing formulaic and overly rigid.

The seven stages of problem-solving treatment represent discrete steps in either the treatment process (i.e. treatment explanation and evaluation of progress) or steps in the problem-solving process (i.e. identifying problems, clarifying problems, setting achievable goals, generating solutions, and then implementing solutions). A detailed understanding of the stages of problem-solving is the key to delivering a successful problem-solving treatment. The seven stages of problem-solving are summarized in Box 3.1.

Box 3.1 The seven stages of problem-solving treatment

1. Explanation of the treatment and its rationale.
2. Identification, definition, and breaking down of the problem.
3. Establishing achievable goals.
4. Generating solutions.
5. Evaluating and choosing the solution.
6. Implementing the chosen solution.
7. Evaluating the outcome after the solution has been implemented.

Stage one: explanation of the treatment and its rationale

It is important with problem-solving treatment, as with any other psychological or pharmacological intervention, to ensure that the patient understands what the treatment is and how it is going to help them. For this reason, it is essential that the therapist provides a complete explanation, in terms that the patient can understand, of the rationale for problem-solving treatment. A direct link should be made between the patient's symptoms, their problems, and the role problem-solving skills can play in problem resolution. This process of explanation can help the patient determine whether the treatment is one that they wish to undertake.

Many patients like the practical approach to treatment offered by problem-solving. In particular, patients like acknowledgement of the link between their problems and their symptoms. The explanation of psychological symptoms, as resulting from problems the patient is experiencing, often accords with the patient's own view of stress and how it affects them. This explanation of how problem-solving treatment works contrasts with the rationale for psychotropic medication which patients are often reluctant to take for a variety of reasons, not least the fact that they usually see their psychological symptoms as being linked to practical, psychosocial factors which they perceive as not likely to be helped by pills.

Although patients may be happy to accept a talking treatment for their psychological problems, many will not necessarily expect the problem-solving approach. Patients might have had previous experience of a less structured psychological treatment, or have discussed such treatments with friends or family. They might be expecting a treatment that will explore in more detail their past and involve discussion of past relationships. They may assume a longer duration of treatment, rather than the brief time-limited problem-solving treatment. Patients may not wish to be the active participants in treatment that problem-solving demands. It is important, therefore, right at the start of treatment, to provide a clear explanation and rationale for the treatment. This will not only enable the patient to understand what the treatment is and how it will work, but also will enable the patient to decide whether this approach to treatment is

Box 3.2 **Explanation of problem-solving treatment**

1. The patient's symptoms are caused by the problems that they are experiencing in their lives.
2. If the patient's problems can be resolved, their symptoms will improve.
3. Problem-solving treatment offers a structured and organized approach to resolving the problems.

one that they wish to pursue. An understanding of the treatment is likely to facilitate compliance. The explanation for the rationale of problem-solving treatment is set out in Box 3.2.

The message that symptoms are caused by problems and that if the problems can be resolved, symptoms will be improved, is one which has face validity for most patients. Patients may be less clear about the third step, namely that problems are likely to be resolved through problem-solving treatment. They will often say that they have tried to solve the problems on their own. The message that the therapist has to convey is that although, indeed, problems may seem very difficult, and the patient may have tried to resolve them themselves, what is new is a chance to work through the problems with someone else. The therapist is someone from outside who may be able to assist with alternative ways of looking at the problems, alternative solutions, and alternative ways of achieving solutions. The patient at this stage does not need to have a detailed understanding of what problem-solving treatment involves but does need to understand an outline of how the treatment is expected to work.

A key task is to motivate the patient to comply with treatment. This motivation is more likely to be achieved if the patient recognizes that the therapist has listened to and understood their difficulties, and has used this understanding to explain the principles of problem-solving clearly and simply. A typical introduction may proceed as follows:

> 'Unresolved problems in our lives can cause us to feel down or blue. They can make us feel like our life is getting out of control and overwhelming us. Problem-solving treatment is a systematic method for learning to clarify

our problems and find solutions for them. As we start to make progress on solving our problems, we start to feel more in control of our lives, and with this increased feeling of control we start to feel an improvement in our mood. Improvement follows action, so we will put a lot of emphasis on having definite tasks for you to work on, at home, between visits.'

There are four detailed steps in stage one of problem-solving treatments. These follow the initial explanation to help ensure that the patient understands what problem-solving treatment involves. The four steps are:

1. Recognition of psychological symptoms.
2. Recognition of problems.
3. Acceptance of the link between psychological symptoms and problems.
4. Practical details of the treatment.

Stage one of problem-solving treatment not only provides patients with an explanation and rationale for treatment but also starts the problem-solving process itself.

Step 1: recognition of psychological symptoms

The first step is to obtain an account of the patient's symptoms. Symptoms can be emotional or physical. Common emotional symptoms include low mood, tearfulness, loss of enjoyment in life, worries, guilt, hopelessness, poor concentration, and irritability. Common physical symptoms include appetite change, tiredness, sleep disturbance, headaches, and non-specific aches and pains. The patient needs an explanation that these symptoms, both emotional and physical, are as a result of their psychological illness, be it stress, anxiety, or depression.

The rationale of treatment rests upon the establishment of a shared understanding that the symptoms are psychological in origin rather than caused by a physical illness. Many patients readily accept this. It is not difficult for the patient experiencing the common emotional symptoms (e.g. low mood, tearfulness, loss of enjoyment in life, negativism, hopelessness, poor concentration, irritability) to accept a psychological basis to their symptoms. However, for patients bothered more by physical symptoms (e.g. loss of appetite, tiredness, sleep problems, headaches, malaise, and aches and pains), the connection

Box 3.3 What the patient needs to understand about symptoms

- What symptoms are.
- The therapist understands their symptoms.
- Symptoms are psychological in origin and not caused by a physical illness.

may not be immediately understood. If the patient does not accept that their physical symptoms have a psychological origin, further explanation by a physician or family doctor may be needed before problem-solving treatment can start.

This step is completed once the therapist has obtained a list of the patient's symptoms. This should have been done in a sympathetic way so that the patient and therapist have started to build up the trusting relationship necessary to underpin the problem-solving process. The patient should have an understanding of symptoms as set out in Box 3.3. This can be clarified as necessary by the therapist.

Step 2: recognition of problems

Once the patient's symptoms have been identified, the second step is to list the patient's problems. The patient should be asked what current problems they have. The therapist may begin by stating:

> 'Now that you know what is causing your symptoms and how problem-solving may help, we should start to apply the problem-solving treatment so that we can help you start feeling better. Obviously in order for you to solve your problems we need to get a sense of what sorts of problems you are dealing with and where to begin. Also, I very quickly get to know an awful lot about a person as we review the various problems in their lives. So, what are the problems bothering you right now?'

The patient should be encouraged to talk freely about areas of difficulty in their lives but not go into too much detail at this stage. What is required is a broad overview of the potential problem areas. The skill is to ensure that the patient has the chance to consider all areas of potential difficulty but without getting bogged down in detail.

Begin drawing up the problem list by asking for a spontaneous report of problems. This allows some indication of perceived priorities in the patient's life. However, do not assume that the patient will spontaneously list all relevant problems. They may not be conceptualizing certain situations as being problems, or they may be forgetting a particular issue, or they may feel uncomfortable mentioning a situation without encouragement to do so. Therefore, it is helpful to ask about any of the areas listed in Box 3.4 that have not been spontaneously reported. For example:

> 'You mentioned problems with work, family, and weight. Are you having any other problems, such as with money? (pause) Your health? (pause) Your husband?'

On rare occasions, the patient may steadfastly deny that they have any problems at all in their life. In such instances the therapist must ensure they have reviewed all of the problem areas listed in Box 3.4.

This is not the moment to achieve great clarity and precision regarding the problems listed. Obtain enough information to gain a working knowledge of the patient's problems but leave more definitive clarification for the problem-solving that will follow. Place the emphasis on getting a broad list of the areas of the patient's life in which they are experiencing problems. Once a problem is mentioned and explained to the degree necessary for a broad understanding, the therapist should ask 'what other problems are you having?' or 'what else?' and move on.

Box 3.4 **Potential problems**

- Relationship with partner/spouse.
- Relationships with children, parents, siblings, and other family members.
- Relationships with friends.
- Work.
- Money.
- Housing.
- Health.
- Legal issues.
- Alcohol and drugs.
- Leisure activities.

Box 3.5 Jill's problem list

1. In debt—£3000 on credit card.
2. Difficult relationship with partner (George)—separate bedrooms.
3. Overweight.
4. Grown-up daughter (Sue) wants help with childcare for grandson (Jack).

The therapist and patient will have drawn up a full problem list by the end of this step. This list will be referred to again and updated during subsequent problem-solving sessions. An example of symptoms and a problem list is illustrated by Jill. Jill, a 60-year-old retired care worker, had several depressive symptoms including tiredness, poor sleep, and a loss of enthusiasm for things she had previously enjoyed. Jill's problem list is shown in Box 3.5.

The problem list does not have to be exhaustive but does need to contain the key problems as identified by the patient and to include minor as well as major problems. It may be easier in the first instance to focus on some of the smaller and more solvable problems rather than tackling problems of many years' standing.

Step 3: acceptance of a link between psychological symptoms and problems

An explicit link should be made between the patient's symptoms and their problems as identified in steps one and two. Patients should understand that their symptoms are a response to their problems. The therapist then explains that the patient can tackle these problems during treatment, and that successful resolution of the problems will lead to resolution of the symptoms. An example of words to use for Jill (the patient whose problem list is given in Box 3.5) could be:

> 'We have set out on your problem list the practical problems you are facing—the difficulties you are having with George, the problems with money, the fact that you have put on a lot of weight recently, and the difficulties that you are having with Sue. In many ways it is not surprising that you are not feeling your usual self with all these difficulties you are facing. I think that the symptoms that you have of poor sleep, not being

able to enjoy things as much, and feeling tired a lot of the time are linked to these problems. What you and I will need to do over the next few weeks is to start tackling these problems. I believe that in working through these problems we will not only help sort the problems out but will also improve the symptoms of tiredness, poor sleep, and lack of enjoyment in life.'

It is important to acknowledge the patient's low or anxious mood, but not to reinforce any hopelessness that the patient may be experiencing about recovery. Whilst unrealistic expectations should not be fostered, some optimism should be engendered in order to motivate the patient.

If the patient following the explanation given in the paragraph above replies by saying 'I have tried to sort out these problems myself but have not had any success and I'm not really sure how problem-solving will help', a response could be:

'It can be difficult when you are feeling down, and also when you fail to sort something out yourself, to see how a new approach will work. I think, however, that if you and I work through these problems together, rather than you trying to do it all on your own, we will be able to make a real difference. I have helped many patients before with similar problems and, although not all of them get better, most find the treatment helpful.'

At this point it is important to emphasize that the patient will play an active part in the treatment. It is not just the therapist who will get the patient better, but the therapist and patient working together that is likely to succeed.

Step 4: practical details of treatment

Once the rationale for the problem-solving treatment has been explained, the therapist then needs to set out the practical details of the therapy sessions. Most treatments are given over six sessions. Initial sessions are one week apart. Later sessions may be separated by two or three weeks. Initial sessions will last an hour. Later sessions may be briefer, depending upon the success of therapy. The patient needs to be able to commit themselves to the full course of treatment before embarking on therapy.

Summary of stage one

At the end of stage one, patients will have been told the treatment rationale and how treatment will be structured. The key points which

Box 3.6 What the patient needs to know

- Problem-solving treatment will be for six treatment sessions over 6–10 weeks.
- Treatment will focus on problem resolution.
- Problem resolution should lead to symptom improvement.
- The patient will take an active part in the treatment process.

the patient needs to know are set out in Box 3.6.

By the end of stage one, the therapist should have an understanding of the patient's symptoms and a problem list. The therapist will also have started to develop a relationship with the patient and will have an understanding as to how readily the patient accepts the problem-solving process.

Stage two: definition, identification, and breaking down of the problem

Choosing a problem

In stage one, the therapist will have completed a problem list with the patient. The next task is to choose one of the problems on the list and employ the problem-solving techniques for the first therapy session. This will both provide an opportunity for the patient to begin potential problem resolution and also introduce them to the problem-solving process. It is necessary to choose a problem that is not only significant and important to the patient but also one which the therapist and patient consider feasible for problem-solving.

Assessment of feasibility for problem-solving is primarily based upon the degree of control that the patient can potentially exert over the problem. Many problems, however, over which the patient may seem to have little control, can be reframed to emphasize those elements which the patient can change. For example, the problem of having to look after three young children under five (which cannot be changed) can be reframed as the problem of having no time to do anything for oneself or no time to do anything with a partner. This is a problem over which the patient might have lost control. Similarly, the problem of having diabetes is not a feasible problem to work on because there is little the patient can do to make the disease go away. However, the problem of having difficulty adhering to the dietary restrictions necessitated by the illness, and which may influence the course of the illness, is more feasible in that the patient can potentially modify their diet behaviour.

The therapist should emphasize that the initial problem chosen need not be the problem that the patient considers the most important. At this stage it should be explained:

- It is important to chose a problem that can be changed.
- More complex problems can be held over until subsequent sessions.

The patient is always the final judge as to which problem to address in each session, albeit with some gentle advice from the therapist. If the patient feels that the problem chosen for the initial work is not particularly relevant to them, they will lose motivation and may comply poorly with treatment. Many patients may wish to make a start on the problem which they feel is most central to their difficulties. The therapist guides but does not choose the problem identified to start the problem-solving process. Box 3.7 sets out phrases to use to help identify the first problem for problem-solving.

Box 3.7 Phrases to use to identify the problem to problem-solve

- 'Which of the problems from the problem list shall we make a start on today?'
- 'We need to choose one of these problems as the focus for this session.'
- 'It's not absolutely crucial which problem we choose for this first session. It's better to choose a problem that you feel we can make some progress with rather than choosing one that is going to overwhelm us. We can perhaps look at a more difficult problem next time or in one of the later sessions.'

Defining the chosen problem

Once a problem has been chosen as a focus for the first session, it should be defined as clearly as possible. The importance of this process for guiding later problem-solving stages, such as solution generation, cannot be overemphasized. In the patient's daily life, the problems are often ill-defined and vague. For example, the problem 'My daughter is rude towards me' is vague and provides no indication of what specifically needs to be changed. Whereas the problem definition 'My daughter tells me to "shut up" when I ask her to do something' is much more objective and specific, and tells the therapist the specific behaviours needing change. It is often helpful when defining a problem to identify behaviours that are a problem, rather than attitudes or emotions. Behaviours are more likely to be amenable to change than other attributes.

In a related fashion, the patient may broadly define a problem theme which is representative of several related, yet distinct, problem areas. This type of problem statement represents not only poor clarity of definition but also a failure to specify discrete problems. For example, a young mother, Anita, reported that she had a problem with 'her family'. On further inquiry, the therapist established that she actually had several different problems with different members of her family. First, she was resentful of the father of her children for not helping enough. Second, she felt criticized by her mother about the quality of her housework. Finally, she had to help with the care of an ungrateful sister with a chronic medical illness. The therapist and patient separated out the separate components of the problem of 'my family' and then the patient selected one specific problem to work on initially.

Patients may describe a complex problem for which the solution is dependent upon multiple smaller problem areas being resolved. The clarity of the problem statement is not an issue, but the complexity of its resolution may be great. For example, a middle-aged, disabled man stated that he needed money to buy Christmas presents. Further exploration revealed that the lack of free cash was related to other problem areas. First, his income was low. Second, he had too many expenses. Third, he was paying off back debt. Finally, he lacked agreement with his spouse on where money should be spent. Each of these problem areas was then established as a target for intervention in itself.

The use of clear and specific language helps with problem definition. Successful problem-solvers tend to translate difficult and vague terms into simpler and more concrete language (Nezu *et al.* 1989). For example, the patient who comes for treatment with 'relationship problems' may feel overwhelmed by this broad and all-encompassing failure, whereas a specific problem such as 'a recent break up with a girlfriend has left me feeling lonely' is less general and will be more likely to be amenable to the later stages of problem-solving.

In problem-solving treatment, the subsequent stages flow from a clear problem definition. Therefore, emphasis should be placed on stating the problem in a clear and specific manner by gathering all relevant facts (being sure to distinguish facts from mere assumptions), using clear non-ambiguous language, and establishing objective behaviours for the problem. The therapist and patient must sufficiently explore the problem to ensure that they both understand and agree on its nature and specifics. In specifying the problem, it may help if the patient considers the following four questions:

1. What is the problem?
2. When does the problem occur?
3. Where does the problem occur?
4. Who is involved in the problem?

If we return to Jill's identified problems listed in Box 3.5 (page 46), there would be advantages and disadvantages to working with any of her four problems. We can consider each in turn. The problem of debt will depend very much on the financial background of the patient. For some patients, £3000 of debt is something that can be easily resolved and yet, for others, it may be an overwhelming amount, many times their monthly disposable income. The debt may already be decreasing or may be increasing. The patient may be spending money in an attempt to cheer themselves up, and this is a recent phenomenon that can be easily curtailed. By contrast, the patient's fixed outgoings may be greater than their income and debt reduction is unlikely to be easily achieved. Although common sense and personal experience often suggest that debt reduction is a rather joyless task, some patients find it very satisfying to gain control over their finances in a structured and ordered way.

A difficulty with a partner is a common problem raised in problem-solving treatment. There is always the concern that satisfactory resolution of relationship issues requires both parties to acknowledge the difficulties and be prepared to work towards resolution. In problem-solving treatment, the therapist sees only one of the couple and inevitably hears only one side of the problem. It is not immediately clear whether Jill's relationship difficulties are longstanding and possibly intractable, or a recent phenomenon which may be linked to a specific cause or change in behaviour. It may be that the relationship difficulties are linked to depressive symptoms (e.g. irritability and/or loss of libido). More information is needed as to the nature of the difficulties. Is the problem frequent arguments and, if so, what are they about? Is anyone else involved? Is the problem simply the couple drifting apart because of other commitments on their time? Jill needs to be helped in clarifying what is meant by a 'difficult relationship'.

Many patients have concerns about their weight and physical appearance. Most of these patients will have tried diets and exercise regimes in an attempt to change their appearance, with varying degrees of success. Short-term goals for weight loss can often be set and achieved, but the patient will know from experience that maintenance of such weight loss can be difficult. Again, weight gain might be linked to a depressive disorder or be part of 'comfort eating' because of Jill's other problems.

Relationship problems with parents, siblings, or offspring are also common difficulties that patients raise in problem-solving. It is not clear from Jill's brief description of the problem what the issues are and where potential problems and solutions might arise. As with Jill's relationship with her partner, more information is required to clarify the nature of the problem.

The choice of which problem to work on first, as already stated, should be left to the patient. In the example chosen, Jill indicated that the first problem she wished to tackle was problem four—that is, the difficulties she was having with her grown-up daughter, Sue, about childcare arrangements for her grandson, Jack. When discussing the different problems, Jill informed the therapist that although there had been relationship difficulties for some time with her partner, the more immediate cause of her distress was friction with her daughter. The patient and therapist were able to further define the problem.

This problem was clarified as 'Sue (the daughter) wants me to look after Jack (the grandson) in the evenings so she can return to work'. Further definition of this problem is set out in Box 3.8.

This example shows how a broad problem can be clarified and defined into a more specific problem. It also shows how the problem-solving process helps elicit important background information relevant to resolving the identified problem.

Box 3.8 Jill's problem

Initial problem

Grown-up daughter wants me to help with childcare for grandson

Further information

◆ Daughter (Sue)	Single parent. Lives nearby (10-minute drive). Wants to return to work—part-time nurse. Has day-care nursery but may have to do evening and night shifts.
◆ Grandson (Jack)	18 months old. 'A handful'. 'A bit spoilt'.
◆ Jack's father	Helps with childcare. 'Not reliable'.
◆ Patient (Jill)	Wants to help out but not sure if it will work. Sue wants commitment to be available for evening and night shifts but Jill has own activities in evening. Feels guilty. Dislikes friction with daughter. Her partner, George (together for past 5 years), does not get on with Sue.

Defined problem

Sue wants me to look after Jack when she is on evening and night shifts. Sue upset because I haven't immediately agreed.

Symptoms as problems

Sometimes patients will mention anxious or depressive symptoms (e.g. problems with energy, sleep, or motivation) as problems that they wish to address. Although these symptoms are 'problematic', they are not objective life problems and, therefore, are not the best problems to identify for the problem-solving process. Nonetheless, if the patient insists that they wish to address these, or there are no objective life problems that appear to exist, then a symptom may be chosen as the problem.

There are ways to fit symptoms into the problem-solving process. The problem definition may be formulated in reference to the functional impairment rather than the symptom. For example, low energy may have the function of decreasing the patient's ability to do housework, in which case the problem definition becomes 'trouble getting housework done'. Likewise, lack of motivation may interfere with going out of the house to visit friends, and the problem definition becomes 'difficulty getting out of the house to visit friends'. As the patient becomes more effective in resolving these functional problems, their depression will begin to lift and the underlying symptoms of low energy and motivation will improve.

Difficulty getting to sleep may be a problem that can be helped by the problem-solving process. Further exploration of the problem of not sleeping might help the patient to identify the precise nature of the problem. It may be, for example, that the patient has found it difficult to sleep and so is going to bed later, catnapping during the day because of tiredness, and then being unable to sleep again in the evening. In this case the problem might be 'I have started to have a brief nap in the early evening and then I can't get off to sleep at bedtime'. Further advice about sleep is provided in Chapter 5.

A summary of what the patient needs to know at the end of the second stage is given in Box 3.9.

The therapist should have tried, as far as possible, to have developed with the patient, a problem definition that is likely to be helped by the problem-solving process. The therapist will be aware of the other problems on the patient's problem list and should keep them in mind should the initial problem chosen cause difficulties further down the problem-solving process.

Box 3.9 What the patient needs to know about problem definition

- One problem has been chosen by the patient to be the focus for the session.
- The chosen problem has been defined, and both patient and therapist are clear what the problem is.
- The chosen problem will be the focus of the subsequent problem-solving stages.
- Other problems may be chosen to be the focus in subsequent sessions.

Stage three: establishing achievable goals for problem resolution

Once the problem has been defined and clarified, the next stage is to choose one or more achievable goals. The importance of having made a clear definition of the problem now becomes apparent in that vague definitions will interfere with setting realistic and achievable goals. This stage is key to successful problem resolution and involves three concepts:

1. What does the patient want to achieve?
2. What is a goal?
3. What is achievable?

What does the patient want to achieve?

An understanding of what the patient wants to achieve involves establishing what, in particular, the patient would like to see changed about the problem. For example, the young mother who had problems with her family (page 50) wanted to spend more time out of the house with friends, and the disabled man (page 51) who needed money to buy Christmas presents wanted to decrease the amount of money he was spending.

It is crucial to elicit from the patient what it is that *they* wish to achieve. This will become important if, in later sessions of

Box 3.10 Phrases to use to elicit goals

- 'What do you want to do about the problem?'
- 'What do you want to change about the problem?'
- 'What would help you feel better about the problem?'
- 'What would make a difference?'
- 'What would make you feel better?'

problem-solving, there are problems with poor motivation and compliance. Should this occur it is helpful to be able to emphasize that the goals were set by the patient and not by the therapist. The clarification as to what the patient's goals are is a key moment in that the patient moves from a consideration of problems to a consideration of solutions. Patients with marital problems, for example, often find it easy to spend a considerable amount of time discussing, at length, their partner's shortcomings and the difficulties that this causes for them, but find it much more difficult to set out specifically what they want to do about it and what behaviours they would like to change.

Useful phrases to use when questioning patients to elicit achievable goals are given in Box 3.10.

If we carry on looking at Jill's problem, the therapist could phrase the question as follows:

> 'So we have agreed that the problem is that Sue wants you to look after Jack when she is nursing during the evening or at night and is upset with you because you have not immediately agreed. What is it that you want to do to sort this out?'

If Jill indicates that she does not know, the question can be asked:

> 'What would make you feel better about the problem with Sue?'

The role of the therapist is to help the patient identify their own goals and to avoid setting goals for them, however tempting this may be.

What is a goal?

The goal is what the patient wants to achieve. Such goals should be SMART goals, as defined in Box 3.11.

Box 3.11 **Achievable goals are SMART goals**

SMART goals should be:

- Specific—clear definition of what the goal is.
- Measurable—it can be clearly determined whether or not the goal has been achieved.
- Achievable—self-explanatory, but considered further below.
- Relevant—goal is linked to the problem.
- Timed—timescale by which the goal will be achieved.

The production of SMART goals is closely linked to the eventual success of the problem-solving process. Once the patient has set a goal, it can be helpful to then ask them whether they think the goal is SMART. An example of this is set out in Box 3.12.

Box 3.12 **John's problem**

Problem

My wife and I are not spending enough time together.

Initial goal

I want to spend more time doing things with my wife.The therapist checks out whether this is a SMART goal:

- Specific—not a particularly specific goal. What does the patient mean by 'doing things?' This needs to be further clarified.
- Measurable—'more time' is not specific enough. How much? How often?
- Achievable—needs to be checked out. Does the wife want to spend more time with the patient?
- Relevant—goal is clearly linked to the problem identified.
- Timed—there is no time by which the goal needs to be achieved.

SMART goal

I want to go out with my wife, just the two of us, one evening next week before the next therapy session.

All goals must have a timescale—short, medium, or long term. Initially, goals should be identified that can be achieved in the short term, for example, before the next session. Medium-term goals can be set early in treatment with the aim that they be attained in stages over the course of treatment. Long-term goals will require continued effort after the conclusion of treatment. Therefore, although long-term goals may be identified in treatment, they will only be addressed via short- and mid-term goals during the course of treatment, and then discussed again towards the end of treatment as planning for post-treatment takes place.

An example of short, medium, and long-term goal setting was a patient who identified dissatisfaction with her career as a receptionist. She indicated that she wanted to become a midwife. It was clearly not going to be possible over six problem-solving sessions to turn a receptionist into a fully fledged midwife, even if she had all the relevant qualifications and experience, which was not the case in this example. Hence, although the long-term goal of becoming a midwife was identified, a medium-term goal was set as achieving relevant qualifications, and a short-term goal, to be achieved before the next session, was to identify what these qualifications were. By the end of treatment, the patient had enrolled in two relevant evening classes. Whether or not this resulted in her achieving her eventual goal of becoming a midwife is not known. She had, however, taken steps to achieve a longstanding ambition. In the process of this, the symptoms which led to her initial consultation improved.

If we return to the example of Jill, she identified both short- and medium-term goals. The medium-term goal was to come to some arrangement with Sue so that she could agree to look after Jack on one or two specific evenings a week. This would enable her to plan her other activities around this childcare. Jill's short-term goal was to arrange a meeting with Sue before the next therapy session in order to discuss how they could come to an agreed way forward.

As with the problem definition, the emphasis is on establishing a clear, defined goal. However, the goal should not be stated in such detail that it generates only one solution and prematurely aborts the solution generation process (e.g. my goal is to go to the cinema next Tuesday evening to see the latest Bond film). Such a specific goal leaves little opportunity for the next stage of problem-solving: the brainstorming of potential solutions.

Another example was Paul, whose problem was that he was not going out in the evening. He wanted to set as a goal, visiting his brother once a week. This is a clear goal but rather limited. An agreed better achievable goal was going out twice a week, once alone and once in company. This leaves open a much greater range of options for the next stage of problem-solving. If a solution is so obvious that it can be generated as both the goal and the sole solution, then the problem probably does not require a problem-solving process at all. The patient should be directed to simply enact the solution and to go on to another problem. The best achievable goals allow for a range of possible solutions.

What is achievable?

It can be difficult for the therapist to be clear about what is achievable within the particular circumstances of the patient, and hence must be guided by the patient. The patient is the expert in their circumstances and their lives. However, depressed patients may be rather negative about what can realistically be achieved. By contrast, patients who are unrealistically optimistic will set themselves up to fail and this will not help the problem-solving process. The therapist must use common sense and the available information about the patient's resources, skills, and support in helping the patient determine whether or not a particular goal is achievable.

What is likely to be achievable is, for both patient and therapist, an area of uncertainty. There is a danger that in order to ensure the chosen goal is achievable, it will be set at too low a level. If this is the case, firstly the goal may not be sufficiently challenging to help resolve the problem and, secondly, the sense of achievement if the goal is achieved is not likely to be great. A simple example of where the goal, although achievable, was not sufficiently challenging would be in the case of a patient who wants to change their job. A SMART goal was identified as 'to draw up a list of possible alternative jobs before next week'. This goal, although both SMART and achievable, is not particularly challenging. A better SMART and achievable goal would be 'identify and seek information about three possible alternative jobs by next week'.

Box 3.13 What the patient needs to know about achievable goals

- The patient has agreed a goal that they want to accomplish.
- The chosen goal is the patient's own goal, not the therapist's.
- The chosen goal is a SMART goal.
- The chosen goal, if medium- or long-term, will have generated a short-term goal to be achieved before the next therapy session.
- The goal is appropriately challenging.

At the opposite extreme, setting goals that are unrealistic will simply lead to frustration and a sense of failure. Unrealistic goals may involve setting too great an expectation on the patient or may involve other people who do not want to co-operate with the problem-solving process. The SMART goal set in the case of John (see Box 3.12, page 57) would probably be unachievable if the patient had disclosed during the session that his wife had been to a solicitor and started divorce proceedings.

A summary of what the patient needs to know by the end of stage three is given in Box 3.13.

Stage four: generating solutions

Once an achievable goal has been set, the next stage of problem-solving treatment is solution generation. The patient is asked to generate a range of potential solutions for the goal set. Teaching individuals to think creatively of a range of possible solutions is based on the premise a large number of alternative actions will increase the chances of eventually identifying particularly effective solutions. In other words, the first idea that comes to mind is not always the best idea. It should be emphasized to the patient that they should try to generate as many solutions as possible via 'brainstorming' techniques. Potential solutions should not be discarded or prejudged, even if initially they seem to be silly or unworkable. Teaching patients to think of multiple solutions helps them to become more flexible in their perspective on problem resolution.

There are several important points to impress upon the patient. First, the quantity of solutions generated is important. The greater the number of potential solutions, the greater the chances for successful resolution of the problem. Second, the patient should feel free to combine ideas when practical to do so, and modify them as they develop their ideas. Third, the patient should not prejudge the ideas until the brainstorming process is completed, otherwise they may prematurely abandon a potentially successful and novel solution. Finally, if the patient is having great difficulty developing solutions, they should be encouraged to think how other people might respond to the problem, or to deliberately invent a solution that is blatantly silly (although it should not be emphasized that generating silly ideas is the objective above generating multiple ideas). This depersonalizing tactic often helps the inhibited patient reduce their concern about generating foolish ideas, and therefore promotes more creative thinking and effective brainstorming for the future.

In order to facilitate brainstorming, it is helpful for the therapist to use statements as set out in Box 3.14.

Therapists should steer away from statements such as 'can you think of anything else?' and 'can you think of any other ideas?' as these invite close-ended responses such as 'no', which abruptly halt the brainstorming process.

Another helpful tactic for brainstorming developed by Nezu and colleagues (Nezu *et al.* 1989) is known as the 'Brick Technique'. The patient is asked to think of as many uses for a brick as possible. Patients typically begin with stereotypical uses such as for building or making a wall. The therapist then asks whether they could use it if

Box 3.14 **Phrases to use in brainstorming**

- 'What else can you think of?'
- 'Think freely.'
- 'Don't prejudge.'
- 'Throw caution to the wind.'
- 'What would your mother/partner/best friend/boss say?'

locked out of the house, if they had a window that would not stay open, if they were attacked in an alley, etc. This exercise helps the patient to think 'outside of the box' and they quickly catch on that they should not limit themselves to conventional rules of thinking.

At the end of this stage of problem-solving, the patient should have generated a list of possible solutions for the identified goal. As throughout problem-solving, the patient should lead in identifying solutions. They are the expert in their lives and are much more likely than the therapist to come up with relevant and workable solutions.

An example of the importance of letting the patient come up with their own solutions can be illustrated by the example of Denise. Denise was a 27-year-old clerical worker who had been referred for problem-solving treatment following an acrimonious divorce. Denise reported that she had lost most of her friends following the divorce, she believed they had sided with her ex-husband. She had been to her GP with symptoms of depression. She had told him that since the divorce she had been lonely and was doing very little in the way of leisure activities—all she was doing was going to work and watching television. Denise's GP suggested that she might join an evening class in order to get out of the house and meet people.

Once this stage of problem-solving had been reached, Denise informed the therapist how irritated she had been with her GP. It was Denise's perception that she had gone to her GP feeling very down and his response had been a patronizing suggestion. Denise had identified the problem of being lonely and had set as her achievable goal, going out twice a week. When asked to generate her own solutions, the ones that she came up with were to get a part-time job as a barmaid and to join a fantasy war games club. The therapist would have been unlikely to come up with these particular ideas to solve Denise's loneliness. She had, however, previous experience of bar work and was aware of a vacancy in a nearby pub. She had been a member of a fantasy war games group before she had married her husband and thought this was something that she would enjoy. She also commented that, as most people playing fantasy war games were men, it would be a useful opportunity to meet someone else.

Once the patient has come up with a range of possible solutions, it is acceptable for the therapist to throw in one or two ideas if these seem to be helpful. Such ideas should, however, be in the form of a tentative enquiry, for example 'do you think that 'x' might be a possible solution?' or 'I'm wondering if 'y' might be something to consider?' The therapist may have knowledge about resources and opportunities that the patient is not aware of, and it would be churlish to deny the patient the benefit of this information. Any ideas that have come from the therapist must, however, simply take their place on the list of possible solutions to be evaluated in the next stage. The patient must not feel that the therapist believes that their solutions are in any way preferable to the patient's own solutions. In fact, quite the reverse message should be conveyed. Box 3.15 sets out what the patient needs to know about the solution generation stage of problem-solving treatment.

If we return to the example of Jill and the difficulties that she was having with her daughter, Sue, about childcare for her grandson, Jill identified as a short-term goal to arrange a meeting with Sue before the next therapy session in order to discuss an agreed way forward. In discussion, Jill came up with a range of alternative solutions:

- To write a letter to Sue to set out how she felt and her ideas as to a proposed way forward.
- To telephone Sue and achieve the same.
- To get her other daughter to act as an intermediary.
- To simply call round and see Sue without advanced warning.

Box 3.15 **What the patient needs to know about solution generation**

- Need to consider lots of solutions.
- It is not only obvious solutions that might be of merit.
- The patient is the expert in their problem and is more likely than the therapist to generate successful solutions.

Stage five: evaluating and choosing the solution

Once the patient has identified a number of potential solutions, the next step is to evaluate these solutions and chose one or more to implement. Many patients find this stage of problem-solving straightforward and are able to easily weigh up the pros and cons of each solution. Some patients, however, find this decision-making stage a difficult one, with the potential alternative solutions going round and round in their minds. It is important, particularly for these patients, that the therapist teaches the patient to systematically evaluate the alternative solutions by using decision-making guidelines. Specifically, the patient is asked to consider consequences for the potential solutions by drawing up a list of the pros and cons for each. The therapist asks the patient to think of the advantages and disadvantages, the feasibility and obstacles, and any other benefits or challenges connected with each potential solution.

Effective solutions are those that not only solve the problem but also minimize negative outcomes for the patient and others. As with facilitating brainstorming, it is helpful to frame comments in an open-ended fashion. For example, 'what are the advantages/disadvantages of x?' implies that there are necessarily some of each dimension. Therapists should avoid questions such as 'can you think of any pros or cons of x?' which allow close-ended responses and invite the patient to opt out of this process. In early sessions, the pros and cons should be considered within the session, but in later sessions, as more problems are tackled during the session, it may be useful to ask the patient to evaluate potential solutions as a homework task. The patient should be encouraged to consider whether each potential solution will:

1. Make a significant impact on the problem.
2. Have advantages or disadvantages in relation to the patient's time, effort, money, or emotional distress.
3. Have positive or negative effects on the patient's friends and family.
4. In all likelihood be carried out in a satisfactory fashion.

In starting the decision analysis process, the therapist may ask the patient a general question regarding any major or salient pros or cons associated with any one of the specific solutions. If present, this solution can then serve as a benchmark and point of comparison for the other solutions. The therapist should then ask the patient to compare the solutions with each other, especially those sharing common themes (e.g. ways to bring in money, communicate with another person, obtain needed information). Only by understanding the relative benefits and obstacles in reference to other potential solutions can the patient be in a truly informed position for choosing the best solution(s).

As with all the problem-solving stages, it is ideal for the *patient* to derive their own pros and cons list. However, there are two occasions when it is acceptable for the therapist to introduce information. The first is when the patient is overlooking a significant negative consequence, either for themselves or others. This would certainly include a consequence of physical or emotional harm, and may include potential interpersonal conflict, such as with a spouse or a colleague at work. The second instance is when the patient mentioned an advantage or disadvantage earlier during the session, such as during the brainstorming phase, but appears to have forgotten this in the current stage. In this case the patient is certainly aware of the issue and is only being reminded to include it in the decision analysis process.

An example of solution generation and the decision-making process for John is set out in Box 3.16.

Once the pros and cons have been laid out for each potential solution, the patient selects a preferred solution or solutions. Ideally, the solution selected should achieve the stated goals while carrying the least personal and interpersonal disadvantages. Some patients find this stage of problem-solving initially difficult to achieve alone, ruminating about possible solutions without being able to choose one, or overlooking important decision-making guidelines established in the previous stage.

The therapist should use their own common sense about whether the chosen solution will have a significant impact on the goal. As with what is achievable for goal setting, on the one hand the therapist does not want to overwhelm the patient with tasks they do not feel prepared to handle, but on the other hand they do not want to trivialize

Box 3.16 **John's solutions**

Goal

To go out at least once with my wife before the next session

Solutions

	Pros	*Cons*
1. Go out to cinema.	Easy.	I don't know what's on; we don't like the same films; can't talk.
2. Go out for a meal.	Can talk about problems; will be a treat; used to go out a lot.	She is on a diet.
3. Go for a walk at the weekend.	Good to be in the fresh air.	Not very exciting; might be raining; might not feel like it.
4. Go for a weekend break to Paris.	A real treat we would both enjoy.	Not practical by next week.
5. Play a game of tennis together.	Good exercise; could have a drink after.	Might be raining; courts might be booked by now.

Choice of solution

2 or 4—will ask wife.

or even potentially insult the patient's sense of competency by allowing a solution which is barely relevant or blatantly unsatisfactory for making progress on the problem.

The therapist should not emphasize the choice of a solution solely based upon whether it is the most 'do-able'. Although the feasibility of the solution is a definite factor, the most important criteria for choosing the solution is whether it has a high likelihood of achieving the goal. Therefore, the easiest solution to implement is

Box 3.17 What the patient needs to know about solution choice

- Each potential solution has pros and cons.
- Choose the solution that will best achieve the goal.
- Evaluate potential solutions properly.
- One or more solutions have to be chosen.

not always the preferred solution. More than one solution may be chosen.

When the patient chooses a solution without appropriately reviewing the pros and cons, the therapist should bring this to their attention. Likewise, if a potential solution, which seems an obvious choice to the therapist based upon the decision analysis, is left on the drawing board, the therapist should inquire about this to ensure that a deliberate reasoning process was used in deciding not to include it as an option. Awareness of using the evidence to choose the solution should be verified by engaging the patient in a brief discussion and review of the important decision-making information after they have chosen a solution (for example, 'tell me how you arrived at the decision to choose that solution').

Stage six: implementing the preferred solution(s)

Once the patient has chosen one or more of the solutions as being the most appropriate way to achieve their goal, the next stage of problem-solving treatment is to draw up an implementation plan for the solution(s). The therapist can introduce this stage of problem-solving with 'now you have chosen the solution(s), we need to firm up the solution into a clear plan of action'. The implementation plan should be as detailed as is necessary to ensure that there are no misunderstandings as to what should be achieved. The plan should be as clear as a medication prescription. Detailed actions and specific dates, times, etc. should be set out. This stage helps to ensure that good intentions are translated into definite action. The therapist should ask:

- 'What is needed to be done or obtained?'
- 'Where is it to be done?'
- 'Whom does it involve?'
- 'How will it be done?'
- 'When will it be done?'

For example, the young mother, Anita, whose goal was to spend time out of the house with friends, chose to ask a friend (Luke) out for dinner. The following steps for implementation were outlined:

1. Call Luke (as many times as necessary to speak to arrange a date for the next week); start tonight.
2. Make reservation at a restaurant (call as many times as necessary to get a reservation); start tonight.
3. Call babysitter; if not available, ask mother.
4. Make appointment to have hair cut; call first thing tomorrow.

The patient must identify and choose tasks that they feel comfortable implementing; the therapist should ensure that the tasks are sufficient to satisfy the requirements of the solution as well. Sometimes this means that the solution may need to be broken down into more simple sub-steps. A new solution may need to be chosen if the original solution requires an action that the patient feels unable to carry out. In the example of Anita, it might on first glance be thought that the proposed implementation plan may fail if the friend identified does not want to go out for dinner. This, however, had been discussed in the earlier stages of problem-solving and Anita was confident that the friend identified would respond very positively to the request. Clearly, however, a plan such as this does rely on the co-operation of others, and unforeseen difficulties might arise. If this is the case, the difficulties will be discussed in the seventh stage of problem-solving at the subsequent therapy session.

If the patient lacks confidence but wishes to proceed with a particular plan of action, then steps may be detailed so as to specify exactly what the patient is to say, when to say it, and otherwise how to behave.

Thus, the patient and the therapist may rehearse an interview in an unemployment office, a discussion with a spouse, a telephone call about a bill, complaint, etc. By the end of this stage, the patient should have a clear set of tasks that are assigned for completion between treatment sessions. These tasks are referred to as 'homework'.

There is a balance to be struck between having an implementation plan that can be achieved by the patient and having one that is sufficiently challenging so that the patient has a sense of achievement having completed it. The two extremes are having a plan that is so simple that it can be completed with very little effort by the patient and is unlikely to have any significant impact on the problem, and a plan that is too challenging and detailed so that the patient will not be able to complete all of it and may have a sense of failure.

If we return to the example of Jill, the implementation plan for her problem is shown in Box 3.18.

Jill felt that simply calling round to Sue's house would be the simplest way of dealing with the difficulties and the way which would make it most difficult for Sue to react negatively. This was based on her knowledge of her own preferences with dealing with conflict and her knowledge about her relationship with her daughter.

The implementation stage is sometimes rushed due to time constraints, as it is the last stage completed during the session. Therapists should be aware that the action steps are the culmination of all the good work that has preceded it. Therefore, to rush through this stage is to lose the value obtained from having completed the previous stages. The successful outcome of the entire problem-solving process rests upon its proper completion. It is well worth the few extra

Box 3.18 Jill's implementation plan

1. Call by at Sue's house in the evening, either Tuesday or Wednesday next week.
2. Take a bottle of wine round—peace offering and a way of easing the conversation.
3. Have prepared what will be possible to offer.

minutes to do this stage well to best ensure a successful outcome for the patient. The therapist must check that the patient:

1. Is clear about their plan—it needs to be written down and discussed.
2. Is happy that the plan is what they want to do to achieve their goal.
3. Gives a clear commitment to the plan.
4. Is aware that homework tasks are crucial to the success of problem-solving treatment.

Once the therapist has drawn up a clear and unequivocal implementation plan with the patient, some time must be spent reinforcing the importance of implementing the plan (that is, doing the homework). The patient should be reminded of the problem-solving process, how their presenting symptoms are linked to the problems identified, and how the problem tackled in the current session is likely to be resolved using the plan agreed. One possible way of explaining this is:

> 'I think that the implementation plan that we have here is a really good one. I think you have done very well in being clear about what you want to do and how to go about doing it. The really important step now is for you to make sure that you do this over the next week. You and I will be meeting only for about an hour over each of the next five weeks. What you actually do between these sessions is going to be as important, if not more important, than what we talk about in the sessions. It's you making a difference to your life in the real world that is going to make you feel better, rather than what we talk about in therapy.
>
> Before we finish the session today, do you have any worries, concerns, or questions about what you need to do before next time?'

Box 3.19 **What the patient needs to know about implementation**

- Clear plan of action which implements the solutions chosen for the goals set.
- Tasks to be completed before next session.
- Homework tasks are as important, if not more so, than what happens in therapy sessions.

Stage seven: evaluating the outcome

The final stage of problem-solving treatment is actually completed at the start of the subsequent session. The patient should have completed or have attempted to complete the homework tasks set in the previous session, and should have recorded the outcome of these tasks on a homework sheet. The therapist begins the session by asking the patient about their success with the homework, 'How did you get on with your homework?', and praising any progress. The therapist can then discuss problems and difficulties, bearing in mind that patients may selectively attend to failures. It is important to praise all successes, however small, without lapsing into a patronizing attitude. For successes, statements such as 'well done', 'I knew you could do it', etc. will suffice.

Praise for achievement should be followed by asking about the impact of the success on the patient's mood. This reinforces stage one of the problem-solving process—the link between symptoms and problems. During the early treatment sessions, patients may state that success in implementing plans had no impact on their mood. This statement may need to be explored further. It may be that the patient's mood has indeed not shifted at all. It may be, however, that the patient did experience a sense of achievement and some lifting of mood following the successful implementation of a task. Although the patient's mood may have subsequently dipped again, the timing of a mood uplift should be noted by the therapist. The therapist should explain that the patient is certainly no worse off for having solved a problem and mood alteration may lag in time a bit. It is important for the therapist to motivate the patient and to encourage persistence. When mood improvement is reported, the therapist should take advantage of this and again point out the link between effective problem-solving and a positive mood state. The patient may be on concurrent medications such as antidepressants. When mood symptoms improve it is important to attribute and emphasize at least equal responsibility to the problem-solving efforts. Attribution of success to medication alone is likely to interfere with motivation and with continued progress after treatment stops.

In discussing failures, the therapist should look for positives in the patient's potential for effective coping. For example, what did they do to try and overcome difficulties. This facilitates a positive problem-solving orientation. If difficulties have arisen, the reasons should be examined:

- Should the goal be defined more clearly?
- Are the goals realistic?
- Have new obstacles arisen?
- Are the implementation steps difficult to achieve? If so, why?
- Is the patient truly committed to working on the problem?

The answers to these questions will guide session two. If the problem is simply too difficult to tackle (usually due to the patient not having sufficient control over the source of the problem), then it is reasonable to go onto another problem or to modify the goal to focus on aspects of the problem over which the patient has more control. It is important to keep in mind that the goal of problem-solving treatment is not to solve all of the patient's problems but to use the problems as a vehicle for teaching more effective problem-solving skills. The important point is that using the problem-solving treatment approach will enable the patient to gain a sense of control over their life and thereby alter their perception of problems, whether resolved in sessions or not.

If the patient has not completed the homework tasks, they may not have understood the central role of homework for problem-solving treatment. It should again be emphasized that progress occurring between treatment sessions is more important than progress achieved within a session. Acting on problems is the chief mechanism by which problem-solving treatment exerts control over mood. The therapist should stress that the goals and solutions were chosen by the patient, not by the therapist, and lead the patient in further discussion of their feasibility. If the patient has successfully completed the homework tasks, then a new problem may be chosen and discussed.

If we return again to the example of Jill, it may have been that Jill's visit to her daughter resulted in an amicable outcome. After an initially perhaps somewhat frosty reception, Jill and Sue might have sorted out childcare arrangements so that Jill would be available on Tuesdays and Thursdays and that Sue would look for alternatives when she had to work on different days. An alternative scenario could be that Sue was not in on the days that Jill went round but she had responded positively to a letter put through the door and they had arranged to meet again the next week. A more negative response could have been that Sue remained very angry with her mother and said that she was going to give up nursing and would not ask her mother to be involved in the care of Jack ever again. The second session of problem-solving would pick up from each of these scenarios and help Jill to work through either the ongoing difficulties with Sue or other issues that she wished to address from her problem list.

Chapter 4

How to structure a six-session course of problem-solving treatment

Introduction

As explained in Chapter 3, problem-solving is a collaborative, structured, time-limited treatment which focuses on issues in the here and now rather than dwelling on problems of the past. The problem-solving process can be broken down into seven stages, the details of which have been set out already. The purpose of this chapter is to provide information for the therapist as to how to structure a six-session course of problem-solving treatment. Much of the information needed for the first problem-solving session is contained in Chapter 3. This chapter will discuss the context of the first session and provide practical resources to support the session. The chapter will then explain how the therapist should organize session two and the subsequent sessions.

Context of treatment

When patient and therapist embark on a course of problem-solving treatment, they may be meeting for the first time. The patient may have been referred to the therapist by, for example, their GP for problem-solving treatment. If this is the case the patient and therapist, in session one, will not have met before. The therapist may have very little information about the patient other than the knowledge that another professional considers the patient suitable for a course of problem-solving treatment. Some information may be provided in a referral letter. Similarly, the patient may have little knowledge about the treatment being offered other than it is a 'talking' treatment.

Chapter 2 sets out the empirical basis for choosing which patients might benefit from treatment. The best evidence supporting the use of problem-solving treatment is for moderate depressive disorders, emotional disorders which have not resolved over a few months, and following an episode of deliberate self-harm. If patients fall outside these broad categories, the therapist needs to exercise some caution before embarking upon a course of problem-solving treatment and will need to understand why the patient and/or the referring professional believes that treatment might be of value. It might be appropriate, for example, that problem-solving treatment is being used as part of a broader treatment package which may include other social or pharmacological treatments. The treatment may help carers identify goals and solutions. Problem-solving treatment can also be used as part of the treatment of patients with personality disorders. It can be particularly helpful for patients unable or unwilling to accept responsibility for their actions and for those who seek professional help but are unclear about what such help might involve. For these patients, problem-solving treatment can clarify goals, the purpose of treatment, and avoid the establishment of a dependent patient/therapist relationship.

Problem-solving therapists may be drawn from a variety of backgrounds. It is not expected that they have particular skills in diagnostic assessment. Some understanding of risk assessment for patients with psychological problems is, however, important. If patients express thoughts of self-harm or violence to others, the therapist, if not experienced in assessing such risks, must have access to an appropriate professional to whom they can make a swift referral. These situations are likely to be rare, but the problem-solving therapist needs to be clear about responsibility and accountability.

Treatment sessions: number and duration

The number of treatment sessions should be explained at the beginning of treatment. For depressive disorders, six sessions is the recommended number of sessions, whereas for anxiety and adjustment reactions, possibly fewer sessions may be required. The first two sessions should be close together (about a week apart) to ensure that the techniques have been understood and correctly applied. The first two sessions last about an hour each and include a detailed assessment of the patient's problems and also an explanation of the rationale of treatment. The patient needs more detailed explanations in these early sessions and more time may be required to establish trust and rapport. Time is also needed to provide the patient with appropriate motivation. Subsequent sessions can be timetabled for 30 minutes. Some practitioners find a 30-minute session rather brief and prefer to schedule in one or two more sessions of an hour before moving to 30-minute sessions later in treatment. It is desirable to apply the full problem-solving technique for at least one problem area per session, in order for the patient to become confident in their use of problem-solving skills.

The problem-solving worksheet

Most of the work during the treatment sessions can be recorded on the problem-solving worksheet (Fig. 4.1). The worksheet can be useful as an aide-memoir for the stages and structure of problem-solving treatment as well as a record of the session.

Early in treatment (e.g. sessions one and two), the therapist takes primary responsibility for recording the information, with the patient following the procedure with a blank worksheet. As treatment progresses, the therapist gradually hands over more of this responsibility to the patient. For example, during session two, the patient and therapist fill out the worksheet together, with the therapist providing guidance. During subsequent sessions, the patient takes primary responsibility for completing the worksheet, with the therapist giving help as needed.

The 'paperwork' can be very useful in problem-solving treatment as it provides a record for both patient and therapist as to what has been agreed in sessions and what should be done between sessions. As the patient completes the problem-solving worksheets themselves, they acquire a deeper understanding of the process of problem-solving than would be achieved simply by talk alone. The therapist needs to make a judgement, however, particularly in session one, as to how

Problem-solving worksheet

1. **Problem:**

2. **SMART goal(s):**

3. **Potential solutions:**

a)	Pros (+)	Cons (−)
b)	Pros (+)	Cons (−)
c)	Pros (+)	Cons (−)
d)	Pros (+)	Cons (−)

4. **Choice of solution:**

5. **Steps to achieve solution (homework):**

a)

b)

c)

d)

Next appointment . . . .

Fig. 4.1 Example of a problem-solving worksheet.

much to involve the patient with the worksheet at that stage. Some patients take an active interest in the worksheets from the start. For others, there could be a perception that the worksheets are somewhat daunting. The therapist needs to strike the appropriate balance between challenging and overwhelming the patient.

Homework

Tasks	When	Progress
1.		
2.		
3.		
4.		
5.		
6.		

<u>Successes</u> <u>Difficulties</u>

Fig. 4.2 Example of what can be recorded on the reverse side of the worksheet.

The back of the worksheet can be used to chart the patient's progress with their implementation plan and can be used by the patient to set out both the difficulties and successes of the previous week (Fig. 4.2).

Session one

The duration of this session should be one hour. If the patient and therapist already know one another (for example, treatment is being given by a professional with knowledge of the patient), the therapist will have a lot of background information about the patient, including demographic information, symptom history, and social circumstances. The temptation when the patient and therapist do not know one another is to spend too much time in the first session gaining this information. The first session of problem-solving treatment is not a diagnostic interview, nor is it the session to determine whether problem-solving treatment is a suitable treatment to be offered to the patient. It is assumed that this will already have occurred. If this is not the case, session one should be deferred until appropriate assessments have been completed, either by the therapist or by another clinician.

It is important that some time is spent in session one in getting to know the patient, as it is part of the rapport-building process which underpins the problem-solving. However, time is limited and much of the relevant information about the patient will come through discussions of the patient's problems. If the patient starts talking about situations and individuals about which or whom the therapist does not know, it is quite legitimate for the therapist to stop the patient by saying 'I don't think you have told me who x is' or 'can you give me a bit of background information about y?'. In this way, both patient and therapist remain focused on the key problem areas to be tackled in problem-solving and do not spend valuable time, however interesting, discussing all aspects of the patient's life.

The following tasks should be completed in session one. Approximate recommendations for the time required to complete each task are also provided.

1. Introduction and explanation of the duration of sessions and the length of treatment (5 minutes).
2. Obtain a brief understanding of the patient's symptoms and background (10 minutes).
3. Explain the rationale of problem-solving treatment (5 minutes).
4. Compile a list of problems (5 minutes).
5. Illustrate the problem-solving process by working through one specific problem (30 minutes).
6. Summarize and confirm subsequent meeting (5 minutes).

1. Introduction and explanation of the duration of sessions and the length of treatment

After introducing yourself, explain the basic framework for treatment. For example:

> 'We will be starting the problem-solving treatment today. We will meet for a total of six sessions including today's session. Today's session will last for one hour to help me fully understand your circumstances. We will then meet for five more sessions of 30 or 60 minutes. We will plan to meet again

in one week from today, in order to make sure you are understanding the treatment procedures correctly. For the remainder of the treatment we will meet once a fortnight. So we will meet for a total of six sessions over the course of nine weeks.'

2. Obtain a brief understanding of the patient's symptoms and background history

The patient will expect to have the opportunity to give a brief account of their symptoms and background. If the therapist already knows the patient, this section will not be needed. It is vital not to spend too long on this subject, however, or there will be insufficient time to do the therapeutic work later in the session. It is sufficient to ask 'how have you been feeling?' or 'what was the reason you went to see your GP that resulted in you being referred to me?' The therapist should identify the patient's main symptoms both in order to track progress during treatment but also to explain the rationale of problem-solving treatment. Avoid being drawn into a discussion of problems at this stage.

It is necessary for the therapist to have a general understanding of the patient's background. This is not the same as obtaining a detailed history. The therapist will need to know something of the social background of the patient—for example, their marital status, their employment, where they are living, what they enjoy doing, and, broadly, what emotional and social supports they have. Much of the relevant detail about the patient's background will emerge when looking in detail at the problems which the patient identifies for treatment. One of the skills of therapy is to keep the general discussion at this point strictly time-limited.

3, 4, 5. Explain the rationale of problem-solving treatment, complete problem list, work through a specific problem

A detailed description of this process—stages 1–6 of problem-solving treatment—is provided in Chapter 3.

6. Summarize and confirm subsequent meeting

At the end of the first session of problem-solving treatment, the patient should have been provided with an explanation of problem-solving, and this explanation will have been developed by the working through of a chosen problem using the problem-solving process. The therapist should ensure that the patient is clear about the homework tasks as set out on their problem-solving worksheet. The therapist should also make sure that the patient is also clear about the date and place of the second meeting. The patient should have had the opportunity to ask relevant questions and to seek appropriate clarification of any issues that they have not fully understood.

Materials to support session one

The first session of problem-solving treatment is a full one. The therapist will, by the end of the session, have obtained a considerable amount of information about the patient. The patient should have experienced an intensive and collaborative treatment in which they feel they have played a significant role in determining the agenda.

It is expected that at the end of the first treatment session, the patient will understand the broad principles underpinning problem-solving treatment, that is:

- Problems result in symptoms.
- If problems can be resolved, symptoms will improve.
- Problem-solving treatment is a way for resolving the problems.

It is unlikely that the patient will remember in detail the structured steps of problem-solving and should, therefore, be given a written handout (Fig. 4.3) in order to reinforce the information that has been provided in the session.

The patient should also receive a copy of a completed problem-solving worksheet (see Fig. 4.1). This will contain the summary information documenting the discussion as the patient and therapist worked on the chosen problem in that session. If possible, the therapist should also keep a copy of this worksheet for review at the next session.

The patient may wish to take a blank worksheet home with them to work on a problem independently, between sessions. This is more likely to occur, however, after the second and subsequent sessions.

How to use problem-solving skills

Depression and anxiety symptoms are very common. They are often caused by problems of living. Problem-solving treatment is a systematic, common sense way of sorting out problems and difficulties. If you learn how to problem-solve, you can lessen your emotional symptoms without having to take pills. In problem-solving treatment, the therapist explains the details of the treatment and provides encouragement and support, but the ideas and plans come from you. Problem-solving will be useful not only now, but in the future, if problems arise.

There are 7 important stages:

1. An understanding of how problem-solving treatment works.
   —Psychological symptoms are caused by problems in everyday life
   —If problems can be resolved, symptoms will improve
   —Problems can be sorted out using the stages of problem-solving
2. Write down a clear description of the problem.
   —What is the problem?
   —When does the problem occur?
   —Where does the problem occur?
   —Who was involved?

   Try to break up complicated problems into several smaller problems and consider each separately.
3. Decide on your <u>goals</u>. Choose achievable and definite goals—SMART goals.
4. List as many possible solutions as you can. Use brainstorming tactics.
5. Consider the advantages and disadvantages (pros and cons) for each potential solution and choose the solution that best solves the problem.
6. Set out clear steps to achieve the solution and indicate exactly what you are going to do and when you will do it.
7. Review your progress and continue your problem-solving efforts.

Problem-solving treatment concentrates on the here and now rather than on mistakes of the past. You should focus on improving the future rather than regretting the past.

Problem-solving may not solve all your difficulties, but it can help you to start dealing with your problems. As your symptoms improve you will feel more in control of your problems and your life.

Fig. 4.3 Example of a summary handout that can be given to the patient at the end of session one.

There is a further handout to be given to the patient explaining in detail what a SMART goal is (Fig. 4.4). The therapist may choose to give out this handout in session one when discussing SMART goals in stage three of the problem-solving process. The information contained is important. However, the therapist needs to be sensitive as to how

SMART goals

The setting of achievable goals is a key stage in problem-solving treatment. Achievable goals are SMART goals:-

Specific
Measurable
Achievable
Relevant
Timed

Specific

Is the goal clear and unambiguous? I want a day out with my daughter is a specific goal. I want to be happy is not.

Measurable

Will it be obvious whether the goal has been achieved or not. I will get application forms for three jobs from the employment section of the paper is measurable. I will look for a job is not.

Achievable

This is in part a matter of judgement and common sense. Saving £10 a week for a holiday may be achievable, winning the lottery is not.

Relevant

The goal must be relevant to the problem. If the problem is increased work because of a colleague's ill health, going to the gym to reduce stress may be relevant, dieting is not.

Timed

A clear plan must be in place as to when the goal will be achieved—by next Tuesday, before we next meet, during the weekend.

Fig. 4.4 Example of a handout, for the patient, that explains what a SMART goal is.

much information the patient wishes to have after one session, and it may be more appropriate to keep the SMART goals patient handout until the second session.

What if the patient does not want to continue with problem-solving treatment

The first session of problem-solving is not when it should be determined whether problem-solving treatment is suitable for the patient. As noted above, this should have been decided before problem-solving treatment starts. However, the patient might decide that problem-solving treatment is not a treatment which they wish to continue with. This decision might have been made by the patient at the time that the initial referral was discussed, in which case the patient will not have attended the first treatment session. However, it will often be the case that the patient will come to the first treatment session with only a hazy idea of what the treatment will involve. The patient needs to be given an opportunity during this first treatment session to clarify not only any issues about the problem-solving process but also whether the treatment is one that they feel happy to continue with.

If the patient seems uncomfortable with, resistant to, or even hostile to the process, the therapist needs to check out whether the patient does in fact wish to continue with both the initial session and any subsequent planned sessions. This should not be done in a confrontational manner. For example, 'Do you think this is an appropriate treatment for you?' may well elicit the response 'no', reflecting the patient's lack of confidence and optimism about the benefit of any proposed treatment. Using a phrase such as 'I sense that you are a bit uncomfortable with what I have been saying' or 'I'm not sure that this is the treatment you were expecting' provides the patient with the opportunity to voice any fears or concerns that they have. These concerns may be allayed by the therapist, or the patient and therapist may agree that problem-solving treatment is not the solution. It is preferable for the patient to be able to voice concerns they have about the treatment rather than simply missing subsequent treatment sessions or avoiding playing their part in the problem-solving process.

Session two

Session two should take place approximately one week after the first session. It is important to have the second session fairly soon after the first session in order to achieve a sense of momentum. It is also important, however, that the patient has had sufficient time to complete the homework tasks set in session one. Session two is usually scheduled for 60 minutes but can be less depending on the complexity of the patient's presentation and therapist and patient preference. Session two is the first time the patient experiences the seventh stage of problem-solving: evaluation.

The tasks for this session are to:

1. Review the patient's progress and reinforce success.
2. Understand difficulties that might have arisen.

3. Support the patient.
4. Address a new problem using the problem-solving process.
5. Guide the patient in acquiring and using problem-solving skills.
6. Set homework tasks.

1. Review patient's progress and reinforce success

The therapist introduces the session by asking the patient how they are. It is important, however, not to dwell in detail at this stage on the patient's current symptoms. Problem-solving is a time-limited treatment and the focus of treatment is on the activities needed to resolve problems. The second question to be asked should be 'How did you get on with your homework tasks?' This leads to the review of progress with the homework tasks. Following this review, there should be an opportunity to link the patient's current symptoms, or their symptoms during the week, with the progress they made with the tasks. Evaluation of progress is the seventh stage of problem-solving and a more detailed description of this is given in Chapter 3. If, for example, the patient set themselves the task of removing the wallpaper from the dining room in preparation for redecorating, the therapist needs to link whether doing the activity led to an improvement, albeit perhaps a temporary one, in the patient's symptoms. Activity and achievement often do lead to symptom improvement and it is important to make this link explicit for the patient.

The therapist should keep in mind that the key to successful treatment is not necessarily to resolve the patient's problems but rather to motivate the patient into taking an active role in overcoming their difficulties. It is often this activity, both the actual doing of the task and also the planning and feeling in control, that will make the patient feel better. Patients with psychological symptoms often feel beset and overwhelmed by their problems. A key to problem-solving success is to counter this by making the patient believe they can do something about their difficulties and by getting them to actively do something.

Self-reward may be suggested to reinforce success; for example, going to the movies (an enjoyable activity) after success in achieving a difficult goal (such as a stressful meeting with a relative).

If the homework tasks have been completed according to plan and the patient wants to move on to looking at another problem, the therapist can, at this point, consider a new problem. If, however, difficulties have arisen, these need to be understood in order for them to be overcome.

2. Understand difficulties that might have arisen

It is common for homework tasks not to go completely smoothly. Several difficulties may have arisen, and these need to be discussed in a non-judgemental way. Clear responsibility for working through the difficulties must be given to the patient, rather than always accepting initial explanations that the difficulties were outside the patient's control. Potential issues that may arise include:

- Patient not undertaken homework tasks.
- Patient partially completed homework tasks.
- Unforeseen obstacles or difficulties.
- Patient has completed tasks but feels no better.

Patient not undertaken homework tasks

It is not unusual for patients not to have undertaken homework tasks between the first and second session. There may be several reasons for this:-

- Patient had insufficient motivation to undertake the task.
- Patient did not want to undertake the task.
- Implementation plan not clearly specified.
- Patient wishes to participate in a less active treatment.

Motivation

If the patient has lacked motivation to complete the homework, the therapist needs to look at ways of improving motivation so that they will achieve the homework tasks before the next session. The therapist can use phrases such as:

- 'What can we do make sure that you are able to do this before next time?'
- 'Is there anything I can do to help you achieve this task before next time?'
- 'It can be really difficult when you are feeling down to find the get up and go to do x but if you are going to get better, somehow we have got to make it happen. What do you suggest?'

This is a crucial and sensitive point in the problem-solving process. It is crucial because if the therapist and patient are not able to work together in order to achieve mutually agreed homework tasks, the treatment is not going to work. Sensitivity is required because it may be that the patient is unable, by virtue of, say, depressive symptoms, to achieve the implementation plan. If this is the case, the therapist does not want to add to the patient's low self-esteem by fostering a sense of non-achievement or add to the patient's sense of stigma by hinting that they could achieve the tasks if they really wanted to. The therapist has to make a judgement whether to persist with the task set, with an expectation that the patient is likely to achieve the task before next time, or whether to explore with the patient an alternative plan which, whilst remaining sufficiently challenging, is more in keeping with the patient's current psychological state.

A common reason the homework tasks have not been attempted is that patients may not have fully understood their importance. The therapist must, therefore, take the opportunity of re-emphasizing that work done between sessions is more important than work done during sessions. It is what the patient achieves between sessions that is going to get them better, and not what is talked about during sessions. Emphasizing this may enhance the patient's motivation to complete the agreed tasks.

Patient did not want to undertake the task

A second common reason that homework is not completed is that although the patient may have understood the importance of the tasks set, they may not have really wanted to undertake them. In this case, the patient has never fully accepted the problem-solving process. The patient may, for example, say that they are not sure that the tasks set were the right ones or appropriate. It is in order to forestall this that during the first session, when problems are identified and goals set, the therapist ensures that the patient leads in making the relevant choices. Hence, if the patient at this point expresses the concern that the goals chosen and the plans set were inappropriate, the therapist should be able to remind the patient that the problems chosen, goals set, and plans made were chosen by the patient and not by the therapist.

If there seems to be no explanation as to why the homework has not been done—'I forgot', 'I've been too busy'—the therapist needs to check out with the patient their understanding of problem-solving treatment and see if they want to work in the collaborative way that the treatment demands. The therapist at this point needs to go back to the problem from session one and remind the patient of the achievable goal agreed. Appropriate phrases to use are 'Can we remind ourselves what the problem was we were working through last time and what the goal set was?' or 'Can we just check out what the goal set last time was?' The patient can then be asked if the goal is still one they want to achieve. This provides an opportunity to either confirm that the goal set was appropriate or, if not, there is the opportunity to set a new and more appropriate goal.

Whether or not the existing goal is still appropriate or a new goal is set, there must be clear agreement with the patient that any plans made to achieve this goal are worked on between sessions. The clear message is given to the patient that they are responsible for the setting of goals and plans and agreeing to them. If the patient shows a reluctance to collaborate with the problem-solving process, the therapist can ask if they have any concerns about the treatment or whether it was the treatment they expected. This will provide the patient with an opportunity to question the appropriateness of the treatment.

Implementation plan not clearly specified

The failure to do homework tasks may reflect the fact that insufficient detail was set out as to what needed to be done, by whom, and by when. This is a failure of the therapist. A new plan needs to be agreed with the patient which sets out the plan in the necessary detail.

Patient wishes to participate in a less active treatment

It may be that the patient does understand the importance of homework tasks and does feel that the tasks set were appropriate and the tasks were clear. However, they have not undertaken the homework because they do not wish to play an active role in getting better. There are patients who visit their doctor in order to be given a treatment that will get them better. They wish to be told what to do or wish to take a tablet that will sort out their difficulties. If this is the obstacle to completing homework tasks, a renewed and careful explanation of how problem-solving treatment is likely to work is necessary. It may be that the patient then agrees that problem-solving treatment might be helpful for them and engages with the treatment with renewed motivation, or it may be that the patient decides that problem-solving treatment is not for them.

There are patients who understand that problem-solving treatment is a psychological treatment, which is their preference over a pharmacological intervention. However, they expect a more psychodynamic or counselling approach to treatment, in which they are able to talk about issues troubling them. These patients may well hope to get some of these issues clarified in therapy and to have a therapist who listens sympathetically but does not require clear action and activity from the patient between treatments. These patients may wish to talk about issues from their past that have been troubling them, such as traumatic and abusive relationships. They may have been expecting that the ventilation of these issues was going to be the content of their therapy. These patients require a further careful explanation of what problem-solving treatment is. Although it may be that the patient will then wish to continue with the problem-solving treatment, alternatively, they may wish to seek another form of therapy which better meets their expectations.

Patient has partially completed homework tasks

The most common finding at the evaluation stage is that patients will have successfully completed some of their homework tasks, but not all. It is important to remember that the patient's low mood may be causing them to magnify problems and failures and to minimize successes. The patient may be magnifying difficulties in implementing solutions and overstating the lack of progress. If this is the case, the therapist should point this out to the patient and praise success achieved. The patient can also be reminded that there are four more sessions after the current one in which to take forward plans not yet achieved—not everything has to be achieved by the end of week one.

Partially completed implementation plans form the basis for discussing problem-solving in this session. This is the bread and butter of problem-solving. The partial successes can be built on and developed. Parts of the plan not yet implemented can form the basis for future tasks. Goals may need to be redefined and solutions chosen with perhaps different timescales and targets.

Unforeseen obstacles and difficulties

Patients are attempting to problem-solve in their real lives, which will continue to throw up stresses and problems that may derail the most carefully laid out plans—a child may have fallen sick, bad weather may have prevented an activity, an unexpected large bill may have stopped plans for a meal out. It is important, when this occurs, to avoid being caught up in the patient's pessimism and lack of motivation but to be clear that problem-solving remains a process that is well equipped to adapt to such difficulties. It can be useful to try and identify what the obstacles are that have prevented a goal being achieved by, for example, going back to asking the questions of the patient:

1. What was the difficulty?
2. Who was the difficulty?
3. Why was there the difficulty?

The patient may wish to attempt the homework tasks again in the week before session three. It may be that the plans need to be altered in the light of new obstacles which have arisen. Alternatively, a new problem may be tackled in session two. The original problem may be put to one side pending more favourable circumstances.

Patient has completed tasks but feels no better

Some patients enjoy problem-solving and get an immediate lift and sense of satisfaction from having completed homework tasks. Other patients get a temporary lift from completing the task which is not sustained. A third group may complete the tasks but feel no better. It is important to pick out benefits in mood if they exist. If they do not, however, it needs to be explained to the patient that it is early days after just one week, that their symptoms have often developed over weeks to months and it is unlikely that they will resolve in days. The fact that the patient is not immediately feeling better is no indication at all that they will not make good progress by the time treatment is completed.

3. Support the patient

One of the therapist's key roles in problem-solving treatment, as in other psychological therapies, is to engender a relationship with the

Box 4.1 Qualities of the therapist valued by patients

- **Listening.** Although problem-solving treatment is a time-limited and structured treatment, the therapist must ensure that the patient's views are listened to.
- **Sympathetic.** The therapist must show an understanding of the patient's difficulties and be perceived as sympathetic to them.
- **Objective.** Patients value an independent assessment of their difficulties by a professional outside their immediate circle of family and friends.
- **Helping sort out issues.** This reflects the content of problem-solving treatment and highlights the role of the therapist in clarifying problems and setting structures for resolution.

patient in which they are seen as supportive, helpful, and trustworthy. Such a relationship is the foundation upon which successful problem-solving treatment is built. When patients are asked about their experience of problem-solving treatment at the end of therapy, most of those patients who feel they have benefited from the treatment highlight their relationship with the therapist as one of the factors which assisted in their recovery. The qualities of the therapist that patients value are set out in Box 4.1.

The problem-solving process is unlikely to be successful unless provided within the context of a supportive patient/therapist relationship.

4. Address a new problem using the problem-solving format

After the review of progress, the remainder of session two should be spent in problem-solving and planning tasks to be undertaken before the next session. These tasks may be linked to the initial problem if it has not been resolved, or to a new problem.

If the initial problem chosen has not been satisfactorily resolved, it may form the focus of session two. The experience of the homework tasks may inform new goals and solutions. It might be, however, that the problem seems to both patient and therapist insuperable and further discussion during session two is likely to be unhelpful. In such a case, it is sensible to address other problems in this session, following discussion with the patient. If a problem is particularly difficult, it may be best to 'park it', acknowledging to the patient that there is a real problem but, clearly, the patient is having difficulties in resolving it at the moment, and both of you have no immediate ideas as to how to progress with it. Both of you can think about it over the course of the next one or two weeks until the next session, and pick it up then, rather than spending all the time in this session focusing on something that may be very difficult to resolve.

In choosing a new problem to work through for this second session, using the problem-solving process, the therapist should review the problem list drawn up in session one. The patient can be reminded of the problems and asked which they would like to work with. The patient may also be asked if there are any other problems that they have thought of during the week that they would like to add to the list, either for discussion now or discussion in subsequent sessions. They must then choose a problem as the focus for this session and work through the stages of problem-solving as set out in Chapter 3.

It may be that the patient and therapist choose not to work through all problem-solving stages in the session but may, for example, stop at one of the stages. This may be stage two—achievable goals; it may be stage four—evaluating a solution. The patient can then be given the worksheet and instructions and asked to work further on the problem at home. If, for example, the patient says that they cannot think of any achievable goals, the therapist can say to them:

> 'OK, it is difficult in the time that we have got now to come up with these ideas, but perhaps if you go away and think about it over the next week and come back, we can pick it up to see if you have made any progress during the week. Meanwhile, I also will see if there is anything that I can come up with during the week and we can pool our ideas next time.'

The therapist can then give the patient the SMART goals sheet (see Fig. 4.4) and remind them exactly what is needed for an achievable goal.

Similarly, if the patient is stuck on choosing the solution, the therapist can say:

> 'I think rather than spending a lot of time on this now, why don't you take this home and list all the pros and cons in the columns provided and come back next time, either having made a choice and drawn up a plan, or having made a choice so that we can then draw up the plan together.'

In this way, a start is made towards more of the problem-solving process occurring outside the therapy session, with more of the process being led and directed by the patient rather than by the therapist.

Another advantage of working on part of the problem-solving process at home is that the patient can seek support from others, if appropriate.

5. Guide the patient in acquiring and using problem-solving skills

In the first session, the patient should have been taken through the stages of problem-solving. They will also have been given a handout explaining what problem-solving treatment is and a completed task worksheet setting out, for a chosen problem, the stages of problem-solving (see Figs. 4.1 and 4.2). The therapist will have very much taken a lead in that first session in explaining and writing down what is happening. In this second session, the therapist needs again to take the patient through the stages of problem-solving but, this time, sharing much more with the patient, as each of the stages are written down on the worksheet. The aim is, therefore, not only to work through a problem using the stages of problem-solving but to be clear and explicit with the patient as each step is being done. In subsequent sessions, it will be expected that the patient will take a lead in writing down the information on the worksheet. This can be explained to the patient so they will know what to expect in sessions three onwards.

6. Set homework tasks

It is important in session two, as in all the problem-solving sessions, that the patient leaves the session with clear homework tasks to be completed before the next session. These should be set out on the problem-solving worksheets (see Figs. 4.1 and 4.2) in order that the homework tasks are clearly linked in with the problem-solving process. The patient should have had the opportunity to ask questions and be clear about the time and place of the next therapy session. If the patient had not been given the SMART goals fact sheet (see Fig. 4.4), this should be given during session two, accompanied by appropriate explanation.

Sessions three through to five

As has been noted, a good patient/therapist relationship is the foundation upon which problem-solving is built. Such a relationship develops over the sessions, and the patient may become more comfortable in talking about difficult issues with the therapist during the later therapy sessions. It is sometimes the case, therefore, that patients bring up new and significant problems in later sessions which were not mentioned when the initial problem list was drawn up. These may be problems which the patient was embarrassed to mention in the initial problem list, or be particularly difficult and sensitive problems such as abuse. The problems raised can be handled in the same way as all problems in the problem-solving process, with the therapist attempting to clarify the problem and, in particular, determining what the patient wants to do about it.

The aims of sessions three to five are to:

1. Review the patient's progress and reinforce success and continued effort.
2. Address problems from the problem list and new problems if they emerge.
3. Consolidate the patient's skills and independence in conducting problem-solving.

1. Review the patient's progress and reinforce success and continued effort

It is hoped that during these problem-solving sessions, the patient will be starting to recover and their symptoms will be improving. This will be the key motivating factor for continued problem-solving. The therapist's task is to link improvement in symptoms with the active working on problems and problem resolution. The therapist should remind the patient of the progress that they have made and of successes from previous weeks to counter difficulties and perceived failures that the patient may describe during the current session.

2. Address problems from the problem list and new problems if they emerge

The patient and therapist should keep under review the original problem list, consider progress, and always be prepared to add new problems to the list. At this point, the patient may have worked through a series of short- and mid-range goals to reach a long-term goal. For example, if the final goal was to secure a new job, the short-term and intermediate goals may have been:

1. To obtain information about the qualifications required.
2. To send application forms.
3. To attend an interview.

For goals such as these, which are achieved in phases, the therapist should track progress over sessions. The patient should be reminded that treatment is time-limited, and hence it is important to concentrate on problems that are:

- Relevant to the patient's life.
- Likely to be helped by the problem-solving process.

3. Consolidate the patient's skills and independence in conducting problem-solving

It is important that the therapist leads by example in the problem-solving process. It is easy to be distracted into discussions of symptoms or unfocused talk about problems. If this seems to be happening, the therapist must remind patients of the limited time that they have in therapy and the need to focus on activities that are likely to be productive in helping the patient get better. It is important that this is not done in an insensitive and crass way, but the therapist needs to be clear that the treatment is more than lending a sympathetic ear to the patient's problems but is to assist the patient in the active resolution of the problems.

In session three and subsequent sessions, the patient should be taking an ever-increasing lead in guiding the content of the session. It would be expected that the patient will be writing out the worksheets themselves and becoming more skilled in setting achievable goals and working through the subsequent stages of problem-solving. It may well be appropriate that whole homework tasks are set in which the patient chooses and works through a problem using the problem-solving framework without this being discussed in the therapy session. The therapy session can then be used to discuss how progress went and to check that each of the stages was accomplished correctly. The patient should be demonstrating an understanding of the skills of problem-solving.

The therapist will need to continue to emphasize that the number of sessions is limited and, hence, the importance of the patient doing more and more on their own. It can help to explain to the patient that many of those who have benefited from problem-solving treatment say that what they liked about the treatment was the feeling that they made themselves better, rather than either having to rely on someone else or having to take medication. This can be a useful way for the therapist to step back, rather than trying to sort out the patient's problems themselves, which may be an ongoing temptation.

Session six—the final session

The aims for this session are to:

1. Summarize progress made.
2. Review knowledge and skills of problem-solving.
3. Anticipate potential or hypothetical problems for the future.
4. End treatment in a positive way.

1. Summarize progress made

The therapist should highlight the progress that has been made. It is also important to review difficulties that have arisen, both those that have proved resistant to change and also those that have been overcome, either in whole or in part. By this session of problem-solving treatment, the patient should have a clear understanding of how the problem-solving strategy will help. The intervention is not a panacea. Six sessions of therapy are not going to resolve longstanding, ingrained problems. The clear message for the patient, however, is that even with seemingly difficult problems, there are areas in which progress can be made. The patient should be reminded that the emphasis is not on difficulties, but what can be done, and also of the importance of identifying what they want to do about a problem, rather than focusing on what it is about the problem that is upsetting.

The therapist should lead off session six with the reminder, 'this is our final session', and then review the problem list and identify any problems that should be considered in the final session. If new problems emerge, the patient should be reminded of the steps they can go through to resolve them, but the therapist should not lead them though a systematic step-by-step approach, unless a new major problem emerges.

If treatment has been successful, the patient should feel convinced that they have contributed to their own recovery, with the use of common sense problem-solving techniques. Achievements during treatment should be summarized so that the patient leaves with a good feeling about the work they have done. If the message regarding the primacy of the patient's own efforts has been delivered throughout the treatment, then problems with termination and dependency should be minor.

2. Review knowledge and skills of problem-solving

This will be the final time that this will be looked at. A review of problem-solving stages should have been an ongoing process throughout the treatment. Clearly, the final session is the last opportunity in which this can be achieved.

3. Anticipate potential or hypothetical problems for the future

The patient can be asked if they are worried about problems that may arise in the future or if there are issues that have not been discussed but are of concern. If this is the case, the therapist has the opportunity to frame the questions within the problem-solving structure and give guidance as to how the patient may move forward should these issues arise. The purpose of discussing potential and hypothetical problems is not to plan clear strategies for resolving them but instead to emphasize to the patient that problem-solving is not something that needs to come to an end once the treatment sessions are finished but, rather, that they have been given a skill that may be used in the future.

4. End treatment in a positive way

It is unusual for there to be a difficulty about termination in problem-solving treatment. The therapist has, throughout, emphasized the time-limited nature of the treatment. The treatment has also placed considerable stress on the patient getting themselves better and working on problems themselves. If the therapist has conducted the treatment appropriately, they will have been more of a guide than a prop on whom the patient has become dependent.

The treatment may not have been successful in resolving the patient's symptoms. In this, problem-solving is no different from other treatments, but this does not necessarily mean that further problem-solving treatment will achieve a positive outcome. It can be difficult for both patient and therapist if a treatment has not worked. The appropriate advice if the patient continues to be troubled by symptoms is that they should seek a further review from their doctor. A decision can then be made as to whether an alternative psychological treatment is indicated or whether medication should be considered.

Both patient and therapist may think, towards the end of treatment, that more sessions would be of value. There is no clear evidence to support this one way or the other. However, problem-solving skills can almost always be taught within the six-session structure. If patients have not been equipped with these skills by the end of six sessions, it is unlikely that further sessions will produce significant progress.

Chapter 5

Other techniques to assist the problem-solving process

Although problem-solving treatment is a treatment in its own right, there are other simple skills that the therapist might wish to integrate into a course of problem-solving. Activity scheduling is the most commonly used of these interventions and will be incorporated into most problem-solving treatments. Specific help with sleep and anxiety can also occasionally be used as part of a course of problem-solving treatment. Care should be taken, however, that the techniques are used alongside problem-solving and do not replace the problem-solving process. If more specialist and specific treatments are needed, it may be that problem-solving is not the appropriate treatment. Communication skills are also discussed in this chapter. Knowledge and use of these skills will enhance problem-solving treatment.

Activity scheduling

Activity scheduling is a strategy for helping patients incorporate satisfying activities into their lives. The procedure is based on research (Lewinsohn and Libet 1972) which showed that depressed individuals engage in significantly fewer pleasurable events that do non-depressed individuals. Lewinsohn's theory of depression postulates that the lack of pleasant events causes the person to become depressed, and because the person is depressed they are less likely to seek out pleasant events. Thus, a downward spiral is established.

The treatment implications are straightforward. In order to help the patient to alleviate their depression, the therapist must help them find and then engage in pleasurable activities on a more frequent basis. The basic tenet of activity scheduling is one that lends itself to problem-solving treatment and is easily accommodated in the primary care setting.

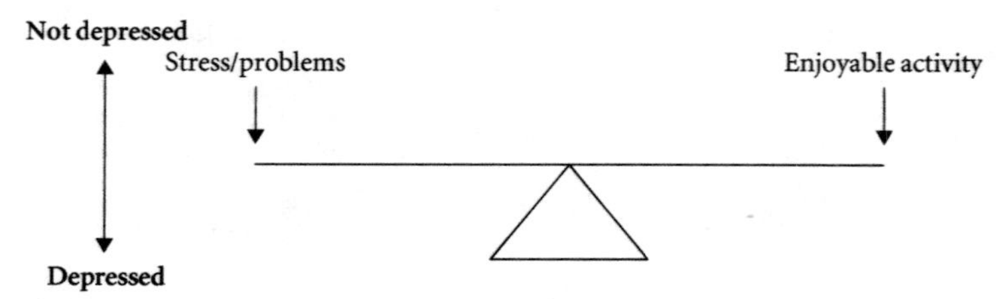

Fig. 5.1 Example of the type of diagram that can be used with a patient to illustrate the balance between stress and enjoyment.

The problem tackled by activity scheduling is that the patient is doing too few enjoyable activities. If the therapist asks the patient how many enjoyable things they have done in the previous two weeks, the answer is often none. The therapist can then explain to the patient that there is a balance in life between stressful events and enjoyable activity. A diagram, such as the one in Fig. 5.1, can be helpful in explaining this process.

If there are no enjoyable things happening, stress and problems can 'overload' the patient, and that explains why they are depressed. Another observation that might be pertinent to the patient is 'You seem to be someone who spends a lot of time helping others and doing things for family and friends but you are not doing anything for yourself'. This can be a helpful way of giving 'permission' for patients to participate in enjoyable tasks. Patients may need specific instruction not to feel guilty about doing things for themselves. The rationale is they will be unable to do all the things they wish to do for others if they remain depressed, and doing enjoyable activities should be seen as a way of getting back to normal functioning.

A role can be found for activity scheduling for practically every patient. Few patients could not benefit from more enjoyable events in their lives, especially if they are depressed. Activity scheduling is particularly useful in the first two or three treatment sessions—the goal of doing enjoyable activities can run alongside other more individual goals. There are several circumstances in which activity scheduling should definitely be used. These are:-

- When the lack of enjoyable events is identified on the problem list.
- When other identified problems are completely outside of the person's control.

- When the solution to a problem is likely to result in increased stress, at least in the short term.
- When the patient adamantly insists that they have no problems to work on.

Activity scheduling begins with a problem definition such as 'too few enjoyable events each week'. An appropriate goal might be 'a treat a day'. An activity scheduling handout, such as the one shown in Fig. 5.2, should be given to the patient.

It is important to stress to the patient that they should identify solutions for the 'treat a day' that they normally would find enjoyable, even if they do not feel like doing them at present. For example, the patient may normally like going fishing but just does not feel any enthusiasm for it at the moment. A helpful explanatory analogy to use may be that of going out to a

Why is it important to do more enjoyable activities?

When people get depressed they do not feel up to doing the kinds of things they typically enjoy. By doing fewer enjoyable things, they begin to feel even worse. As they feel worse, they do even less. So they get caught up in a vicious cycle of doing even less and feeling even worse.

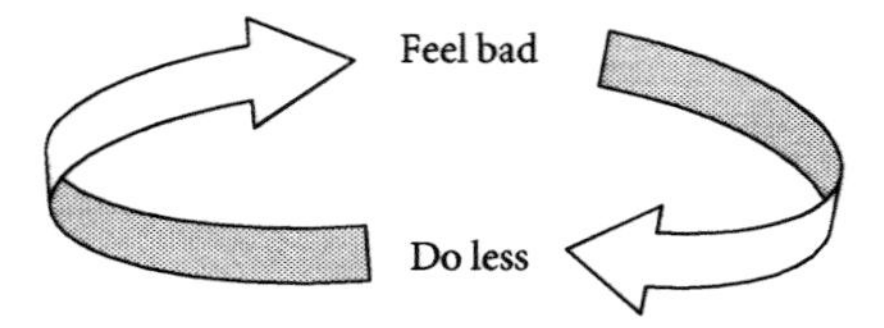

A simple and effective introduction to problem-solving is to take as the problem: reduced enjoyable activity, and to set a goal of doing one enjoyable activity each day. In other words, arranging to provide yourself with 'a treat a day'.

The positive benefits are:

a) You can work through the steps of problem-solving using a simple problem

b) The tasks can usually be easily arranged and managed

c) You will start to assert control over your life

d) You will break the cycle of not doing enough enjoyable activities

If possible one of the enjoyable activities should be exercise or a physical activity—this will benefit your health as well as your mood. Also, if possible, choose one activity that involves meeting someone—a friend or a family member.

Fig. 5.2 Example of an activity scheduling handout.

party—you may not feel like going but when you make the effort it is often enjoyable.

Sleep problems

Many patients with anxiety and depressive disorders describe sleep difficulty. Although this is a psychological symptom, it may be chosen by the patient as a problem which they wish to work on in problem-solving treatment. The causes of insomnia in primary care are listed in Box 5.1. The therapist might want to consider this list for patients with sleep difficulties.

Many patients do not sleep well because of taking part in activities that interfere with the maintenance of good-quality sleep. A knowledge of the principles of sleep hygiene may help these patients. Sleep hygiene is based on a series of common sense factors that identify what might be preventing patients from sleeping. The main rules for sleep hygiene can be set out in a patient information handout, such as the one in Fig. 5.3.

Box 5.1 Causes of insomnia in primary care

1. Depression	Approximately 30% of patients with insomnia have a moderate depressive disorder.
2. Substance abuse	Substances to consider include: Alcohol. Hypnotics. Caffeine. Illicit drugs.
3. Physical illness	Painful illnesses. Chronic medical illnesses. Nocturnal asthma. Movement disorders.
4. Environmental factors	Noise. Temperature. Light.

Rules for better sleep

1 **Reduce time in bed**
- Do not spend time awake in bed (get up, read/listen to music).
- Avoid daytime naps (in bed or elsewhere).

2 **Avoid caffeine, alcohol, and nicotine**
- Low doses of alcohol promote sleep, but as alcohol is metabolized, sleep becomes disturbed.
- Avoid caffeine from afternoon onwards.

3 **Exercise in late afternoon or early evening**
- Exercise is helpful for sleep but leads to over-arousal in evening.

4 **Regular bedtime**
- Go to bed at same time.
- Get up at pre-set time whatever sleep obtained.

5 **Eliminate bedroom clock**
- Once alarm is set, hide the clock away and do not keep looking at it.

6 **Avoid stimulating/upsetting activity before sleep**
- Do not do work in late evening.
- Avoid arguments in evening.
- Set a worry time for earlier in the day.

7 **Get environment right**
- Comfortable bed.
- Bedroom neither too hot or cold.
- Quiet (consider ear plugs).
- Blackout light.

8 **Eat a light bedtime snack**
- Do not eat main meal late in evening.
- Milky drinks may help.

Fig. 5.3 Example of a patient information handout outlining rules for good-quality sleep.

The principles of sleep hygiene can be fitted into a course of problem-solving treatment by taking as the problem 'I'm not getting enough sleep'. An appropriate goal could be to identify and change factors which might be stopping sleep. The patient and therapist then brainstorm reasons why the patient is not sleeping. The use of the sleep hygiene rules may assist this process, but the brainstorming need not be limited to these rules. The therapist will also need to bear in mind the possibility that substance abuse and physical illness may be linked to the sleep difficulty. If this seems to be the case, the therapist might point this out to the patient.

Once factors have been identified that seem to be linked to the sleep problem, possible solutions to change these factors should be identified and worked up into a plan. Thus, the therapist has provided information to the patient about the causes of poor sleep but the 'problem' has been addressed through the problem-solving process.

Simple anxiety management techniques

Many patients treated with problem-solving have anxious symptoms. The usual problem-solving approach to be adopted is that the patient and therapist address underlying problems with the expectation that the anxious symptoms will improve as the problems are resolved. However, some patients may have a particular problem with an anxious symptom that they wish to tackle directly. If this is the case, the therapist may use one or more of the techniques set out below as part of problem-solving treatment. These techniques can be incorporated into the problem-solving process. For example, if a patient is having panicky symptoms of hyperventilation, one of their goals can be to use the breathing or distraction techniques in anxiety provoking situations. Patients who are developing mild phobic symptoms can set as a goal, facing the feared situation for a certain time and on a certain number of occasions. Two simple techniques can be shared with the patient as ways of reducing or helping them to cope with anxiety—slow breathing and distraction.

Slow breathing

Hyperventilation (over breathing) may precipitate anxiety and is often a maintaining factor as patients worry about their hyperventilation symptoms. Patients often describe the taking of deep breaths as a way of coping, and then give a convincing demonstration of hyperventilation. Dizziness and tingling in the fingers are common symptoms experienced by individuals who hyperventilate. Asking a patient to breathe quickly and shallowly for 30 seconds can often convincingly demonstrate the relationship between breathing and

Box 5.2 Slow breathing

- Breathe in for 4 seconds and out for 4 seconds, pause for 4 seconds before breathing again.
- Practise for 10 minutes, morning and night.
- Use before and after situations that make you anxious.
- Regularly check and slow down breathing throughout the day.

anxiety symptoms. These patients need to slow their breathing down. Patients can be given the information set out in Box 5.2 about slow breathing.

Some patients also find it useful to cup their hands over their mouth and nose as a way of regulating their breathing if they have begun to hyperventilate. The same can be achieved by using a paper bag. However, the use of cupped hands is less conspicuous.

Distraction

Patients can be informed that worrying thoughts lead to anxious symptoms, which in turn often worsen worrying thoughts. A vicious circle is thus established, as shown in Fig. 5.4.

Distraction is a method which can be used to empty the mind of worrying thoughts and replace them with neutral thoughts. This will then reduce the physical symptoms of anxiety. If using distraction, patients are advised to:

- Describe in detail to themselves a picture, a view, a story, etc.
- Think of a relaxing image (e.g. the seashore, a lake, mountains).
- Save up worries to a circumscribed 'worry time' each day.

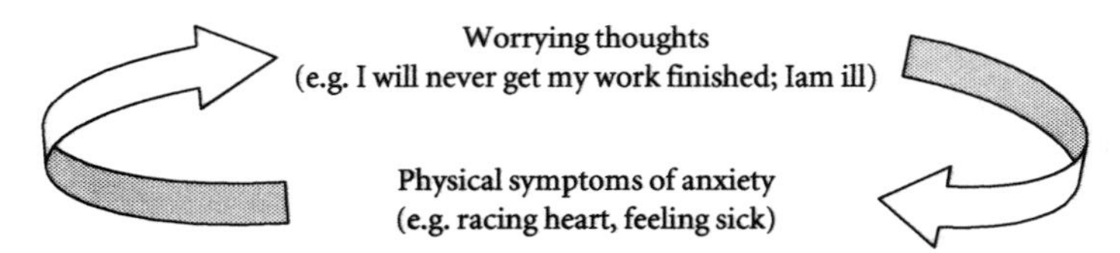

Fig. 5.4 The anxiety/anxious symptoms circle.

Relaxation can be thought of as a distraction technique. If the patient is focusing on tensing and relaxing muscles, or a particular image, it is more difficult to be simultaneously worrying. There are a number of different relaxation techniques and a number of relaxation tapes available.

If the patient identifies as a problem being unable to cope with anxiety provoking situations, the goal can be to identify what makes the patient anxious and what can be done to reduce anxiety. The patient can then brainstorm options, with the therapist adding information about distraction and slow breathing as appropriate.

Simple exposure

Avoiding feared situations is an important factor in many anxiety disorders. Each time a situation is avoided, the idea is further strengthened in an individual's mind that they would have been overwhelmed by anxiety. Patients should be advised to face the feared situation and remain in it until either the anxiety subsides, or until they can convince themselves that being in a situation will not lead to them losing control or being unable to deal with the anxiety. Avoiding feared situations allows the fear to grow stronger, whereas repetitively confronting feared situations will reduce the fear.

The essential feature of exposure-based psychological treatment involves persuading the patient to stop avoiding the feared situation. Patients are told this will initially result in heightened levels of anxiety but will enable them to 'put to the test' predictions about losing control, going mad, etc. Repetitive exposure to the feared situation and a repetitive invalidation of feared consequences leads to a reduction in anticipatory anxiety, avoidance, and disruption to an individual's life. Patients can be given the information as set out in Box 5.3.

Once patients have been given advice about exposure, they can often take themselves through several tasks. In the initial stages, a friend or relative can often assist in the process. However, care should be taken that dependence does not develop or that being accompanied is not an avoidance.

Exposure and response prevention techniques are a stand-alone psychological treatment. For patients significantly disabled by phobic,

Box 5.3 Simple exposure

- Draw up a list of avoided situations.
- Start with easier tasks and build up to harder tasks.
- Face feared situation as often as possible.
- Remain in the situation.
- Experiencing anxiety allows prediction of 'loss of control' to be challenged.

obsessional, or avoidant symptoms, exposure and response prevention is the treatment of choice rather than problem-solving treatment. However, many suitable problem-solving patients have mild phobic symptoms which have developed alongside their other depressive and anxious symptoms. These phobic avoidances may well be causing significant difficulties for the patient and be chosen as their problem focus. In these circumstances, guiding the patient choice of goal to involve exposing them to avoidant situations can be helpful.

An example of this was Mark, who had begun to avoid watching his eight-year-old son (Matt) play football. He had had an argument with one of the other fathers when he had been refereeing a match and was worried this might happen again. Mark had become increasingly reluctant to go to the matches and had refused to be a referee again. Matt's mother was taking Matt to most of the matches. Mark's goal was set as taking Matt to the match but not initially acting as a referee. Mark and the therapist brainstormed options to make this possible and agreed that Mark would go first with his wife and then, if this went well, he would go with just Matt. This was successful and, by the end of the problem-solving course, Mark had achieved a more challenging goal and had acted as a referee again.

Communication skills

Communication skills include questioning, listening, responding, explaining, summarizing, negotiating, and non-verbal communication. An ability to use these techniques will facilitate the problem-solving process.

Questioning

Open questions encourage patients to tell their own story and reveal information that might otherwise not have been volunteered. They are particularly helpful at the start of a discussion and when more information is needed. An example: '*How can I help you?*' 'Well, I really feel awful.' '*Could you tell me a bit more about it*?' 'I feel tired all the time, I cry a lot, and I feel so nervous. I think it has to do with work.' '*Could you tell me . . .*'

Probing questions may also be helpful. These are follow-up questions that stimulate patients to think more deeply about their answers. For instance, in this patient: '*Have you noticed anything that brings on this nervousness*?'

Prompts are questions that contain hints to encourage patients to augment their story: '*You just told me that your colleague is the one causing you to feel anxious. Can you tell me what does she do exactly that brings on your anxiety*?'

Closed questions are likely to produce short answers and are helpful when you are searching for particular items of information such as specific emotional symptoms or problems. This type of question is particularly helpful when you want to determine the presence or absence of a clear mental disorder, for example: '*Do you feel sad?*', '*Have you lost weight*?'

Leading questions should be avoided because they encourage patients to give answers they believe you want to hear: '*Would you agree that her criticisms bring on your tears?*' Also, try to avoid asking overlapping questions as this will confuse a patient and they are very difficult to answer accurately: '*Do you have difficulty with your appetite and weight?*' The answer to appetite and weight may be different. It is better to ask the questions separately and wait for the answers in between.

Listening and responding

Active listening is trying to understand the message, verbally and non-verbally. This means *clarifying* now and then, sometimes *repeating* in your own words what a patient has said and making sure you have really understood: 'There were lots of difficulties in taking care of your mother, you told me you nearly broke down. Could you tell me what you mean exactly? What happened? How did you manage?' It also means *reacting with empathy* when required: 'You had been very close. When your mother died this must have been very difficult for you.'

Summarizing

A summary helps to clarify that all relevant details have been told. If it is done in an appropriate way it will also show the patient that you have really paid attention to their story. The summary can also be used to check if everything was understood correctly, and the patient should have the opportunity to correct or to add information: 'You told me that you took care of your mother for a long time and that was very difficult because she lived 60 miles away. Also you had nobody to support you. Have I understood this correctly?'

Explaining

When explaining to a patient about symptoms, diagnosis, or treatment, make sure that you *adjust your explanation* to the individual patient, building on their existing knowledge. Use words appropriate to the patient's knowledge and understanding. Do not tell too much at once, take your time, and make sure to leave space for questions. Assess the patient's understanding by asking them specific questions during or following an explanation.

Negotiating

In problem-solving treatment, the patient should be the lead decision maker, but the therapist guides the structure and process of treatment. Although, therefore, the patient should identify goals and homework, it is not acceptable for no goals or homework to be set. At times, a process of negotiation is necessary. Listen actively and clarify exactly what it is that the patient wants or does not want, and why. Respond to emotions in a way that makes the patient feel understood, for instance: 'You are disappointed that your doctor found no physical explanation for your headaches, and you would like another scan but your doctor thinks problem-solving might help and be a better option. Shall we give it a go?' Try to reach an agreement about what should be done (or not done). Ask the patient to participate: 'Let's try to come up with a plan we can both agree on. Do you have any ideas?' Sometimes it is important to give the patient (and/or yourself) some extra time or a time-out, for example: 'Shall we take some more time to think about possible solutions and talk about it in the next session?'

Non-verbal communication

Throughout treatment, the therapist should be aware of the non-verbal communication of their patients as well as of themselves. For recognition of emotional distress it is important to make eye contact, to have a relaxed posture, to not just sit passively but nod now and then, encouraging the patient to tell more. Watch the expression on the patient's face, their posture and gestures when they are telling their story.

Avoid giving information too early

One of the skills of problem-solving treatment is to avoid giving advice but rather to facilitate a process whereby the patient chooses from options. The therapist may need to provide the patient with information, however, to guide and assist these choices. Information should be given after the patient has had the opportunity to explain their point of view. Information can then be tailored to take account of the patient's position and is more likely to be understood and accepted.

Chapter 6

Additional guidelines for effective problem-solving treatment

Although the principles of problem-solving treatment are relatively simple, the delivery of treatment is a skilled task. Experience has shown a number of factors to be important in successful delivery of treatment, and these are examined in this chapter.

The patient/therapist relationship

In all psychological treatments and indeed most other therapeutic relationships, the relationship between patient and therapist is important. Problem-solving treatment techniques can seem to be very simple. Indeed, the principles of the treatment are clear and straightforward. The skill of the therapist, however, is to deliver the treatment in a way which takes account of the complexity of the patient and their problems. The relationship in problem-solving is not explored as with dynamic therapies, but the treatment is unlikely to be effective if the patient does not feel confident in the therapist's abilities and assured of the therapist's best intentions.

Research has validated the importance of the therapeutic relationship in therapy. The most significant variable that distinguishes a successful from an unsuccessful therapist is the ability to form a good therapeutic alliance with the patient. Key factors in developing such a therapeutic alliance include trust, rapport, and warmth.

Trust

The therapist's implicit and sometimes explicit messages should be that they care about and value the patient, are confident that they can work together, and are not overwhelmed by the patient's problems. Techniques such as frequent summarizing as well as checking the patient's perception at the end of each session are ways of demonstrating respect for and collaboration with the patient.

Trust implies a two-way interaction between patient and therapist. Patients will only trust a therapist if they know that the therapist can be relied on to try to understand their perspective. It is neither necessary nor desirable to agree with the patient's views, but the therapist must convince the patient that they are making every effort to understand their point of view. Patient confidence and trust is engendered by ensuring that the therapist plays close attention to what the patient is saying. This is a key aspect of problem-solving treatment in which the patient's choice of problems and goals are so crucial. The patient also needs to feel that the therapist is acting in their best interest, even if they disagree on the required action. It is also important that the therapist is reliable and that they keep to any promises or agreements that have been made. Patients rely on the certainty that the therapist will not overstep their professional boundaries and behave like a friend or a relative.

Genuineness is a factor enhancing trust. The therapist should convey honesty, tempered by the knowledge that the patient needs to be supported and motivated. Being overpositive can be as unhelpful as being negative if it is seen as patronizing or insincere.

Rapport

A good rapport allows a disagreement to occur between patient and therapist without the patient feeling judged, enabling the patient to correct the therapist when there has been a misunderstanding. Strategies such as attentive listening, regular summarizing, and a clear attempt to understand the patient's perspective will go a long way to building up good rapport between the patient and therapist. The patient's initial reaction to the problem-solving approach may include statements such as 'It's too simple. I must be depressed for some other reason' or 'I've tried this process on my own' or 'The problem-solving approach seems to ignore feelings'. The manner in which the therapist responds to such statements can convey a sense of rapport and help ensure that the patient will begin treatment with a wait-and-see attitude rather than a sense that problem-solving is not the treatment for them.

A warm attitude and an ability to convey a sense of concern will help establish rapport. A balance needs to be struck between over-enthusiastic warmth and professional distance, both of which, at extremes, can be unhelpful.

Sympathy

The therapist needs to convey to the patient a sympathetic approach to the difficulties that they are having without becoming over-involved. Patients value the fact that the therapist is more detached and perhaps more objective than family and friends, but this does not imply coldness or a lack of interest in the patient's difficulties. The therapist must attempt to tailor the problem-solving approach to the individual patient's needs. This will involve using the patient's own words and language where possible and explaining concepts in a language that will be meaningful to the patient, rather than using rigid and formulaic phrases. It is important that the therapist avoids creating a sense of dependency by suggesting too many ideas or undertaking tasks themselves.

The role of the therapist as teacher

The therapist should always remember that, in conducting problem-solving treatment, they are teaching the patient new skills which it is hoped will remain with the patient well beyond the end of treatment. Instruction in the specific concepts and procedures of problem-solving is as important as helping the patient resolve specific problems in the treatment sessions. The therapist should be conducting an ongoing assessment of the patient's level of understanding and ability to employ the problem-solving techniques, and should be teaching the concepts actively, rather than merely demonstrating them during treatment sessions. Frequent reference to the various stages (for example, 'achievable goal', 'brainstorming', 'pros and cons'), as well as requiring the patient to identify the 'next step' in problem-solving, are useful strategies for assessing and teaching the problem-solving skills.

Regular summaries of the process

During each session, the therapist should make an effort to summarize the problem-solving strategy and emphasize its link to symptom improvement. This is ideally done at both the beginning and end of each session. At the beginning, the summary can be provided in the context of reviewing homework tasks and linking their completion to symptom improvement. At the end, the summary can be provided in the context of reviewing the problem-solving work conducted during the session and the homework tasks set.

Avoid reinforcing irrelevant material

Problem-solving treatment is a highly focused and brief therapeutic intervention. In order to conduct problem-solving treatment properly, it is not feasible to allow much digression from relevant discussion. Patients with previous experience of other, less focused, therapy approaches may unwittingly divert the structure of the session to more general types of discussion. To allow them to do this unchecked will subvert the goals of problem-solving treatment. This does not, however, preclude the therapist from being appropriately supportive when indicated.

The therapist should develop tactful methods for limiting digression. Statements at the start of the session such as 'alright, we have 30 minutes together, let's see what we can accomplish' help to set the tone for a focused interaction. Further into the session, statements such as 'OK, we have 10 minutes left and need to pick a solution for a homework task' is useful for getting a wandering patient back on track. Casually holding up a hand to interrupt the patient and saying 'this line of discussion is very important, and I want to be sure to return to it, perhaps next session, but right now we need to establish the homework tasks for this week' is often effective in redirecting the patient without insulting them.

Moving on when stuck

There will be many occasions when the problem-solving process does not flow smoothly from defined problems through achievable goals and solutions to implementation plans. Patients may have difficulties at any point during this process, and a key role for the therapist is to help the patient through these difficulties. There will be occasions, however, when after appropriate discussion and exploration, both patient and therapist are not sure whether it is possible, for example, to identify achievable goals or identify potential solutions for defined goals. On these occasions it can be helpful to acknowledge the difficulty and move on. Problem-solving is not going to solve every problem. It might prove necessary to choose another problem from the list in order for the patient to experience a sense of achievement in one problem area, even if not the initial one chosen. It is important when this is done that the patient does not feel a sense of hopelessness or that their chosen problem is being dismissed. One way of doing this is to say:

> 'I think we are getting a bit stuck here. I am anxious that we are able to achieve some success in this problem-solving session and wonder whether we should not park this problem for today and come back to it next week? Perhaps you and I can have a think, before the next session, about how we can sort this one out? Meanwhile, we have fifteen minutes left, can we choose another area to look at?'

One of the homework tasks can then be to try and resolve the difficult issue by, for example, coming up with an achievable goal or identifying possible solutions.

Assign parts of problem-solving treatment for homework

For therapeutic and teaching purposes, it is desirable to apply the full problem-solving treatment procedure for at least one problem during treatment sessions. However, it may simply not be feasible to address all the problems and potential solutions within the space of one meeting and, therefore, homework can include the practice of specific problem-solving skills (for example, brainstorming, weighing up pros and cons) in addition to specific homework tasks for problems addressed in the session. By the end of the first few sessions, several problem areas have typically been addressed, and the work related to intermediate and long-term goals will start to add up. It may be appropriate at that point to spend the bulk of the working session on new problem areas and to assign the work related to the long-term problems for homework.

Praise progress explicitly

The reinforcement that comes from successful problem-solving is at the root of the effectiveness of treatment. In keeping with this process, explicit and generous verbal reinforcement (without sounding patronizing) of progress is essential. This facilitates a positive problem-solving orientation and helps establish a good therapeutic alliance. Especially early in treatment, when patients are more likely to focus on failures rather than successes, it is important that the therapist point out and praise successful efforts. At the same time, the therapist should tease out any possible positive impact that the success has had on the patient's mood. Statements such as 'How did it make you feel to have successfully tackled that problem?' are helpful in this regard.

Loop back to earlier stages when necessary

While generating potential solutions to a problem or identifying the steps to achieve a solution, the therapist and patient often discover that the problem is more complex than they initially imagined. If the view of the original problem seems to be getting murkier, rather than clearer, during these stages, then this is a sure sign that the problem statement or the goal needs to be reworked. Do not hesitate to return to the original problem and repeat the early stages of problem-solving. The quality of the problem and goal statements will have repercussions throughout the remaining stages of problem-solving, and time is well spent in going back to redefine the problem and goal definitions. An example of how this process of looping back works is given for a patient, Paul, in Box 6.1.

Paul's problem was debt; his achievable goal was to sell his house; one solution was that he needed to get the house ready for being sold. Paul recognized that his house would need some 'tidying up' in order to get the best possible price and this included sorting out the garden and making some improvements to the internal décor. It became clear, therefore, that a better achievable goal than selling the house was getting the house improved to be sold. By going back to change the

Box 6.1 **Paul**

Paul is a 54-year-old married man with two grown-up sons. He and his wife have significant financial worries and are unable to meet their mortgage repayments. The elder son is in the army and the younger one is hoping to leave home and move into a flat with friends.

Problem

In debt—need to move to a smaller house to release equity and decrease mortgage

First achievable goal

Sell the house

Solutions

1. Ring estate agents for valuations.
2. Need to get house ready for sale.

achievable goal, Paul was able to come up with the following solutions:

- Tidying up the garden.
- Decorating the front room.
- Getting the outside of the house painted.

This second discussion of potential solutions became somewhat overwhelming, and so Paul and the therapist looped back to set a third goal which was more achievable than the second and better than the first. The third goal was to redecorate the downstairs front room (which had not been decorated for some time and had a large stain on the ceiling from when the bath had overflowed). Paul was able to identify the following solutions to this:

- Ask his brother to help.
- Ask his teenage son to help.
- To take two days off work.
- Pay for a painter and decorator friend to assist.

Paul decided that the best option was to ask his brother to help. He then worked through a detailed implementation plan as to how the front room could be redecorated.

This example illustrates how the patient and therapist can loop back through the problem-solving process to come up with achievable goals and eventual solutions that are feasible and relevant. In subsequent sessions, it would be perfectly appropriate, in the example given, if Paul were to choose one or both of the remaining second set of solutions as achievable goals or implemented solution one from the first goal set.

One of the key problem-solving processes is to assist the patient in clarifying problems and goals and to move from broad, vague, overwhelming goals to smaller, more specific and manageable goals. Looping back is an important mechanism to facilitate this process.

Point out major unforeseen obstacles

In most circumstances, the patient should be allowed to choose their own solutions and steps to achieve them. After all, one of the goals of problem-solving treatment is to help patients learn to evaluate their own ideas and actions. Part of the value of problem-solving treatment is in the learning the patient acquires through failed efforts. Although these failures ought not to be directly planned, they do provide useful information for subsequent problem-solving efforts. However, in order to maximize the chances for success, and to limit the probability of strongly aversive outcomes, the therapist may at times point out that a chosen course of action may have a major unforeseen negative consequence (for example, upsetting a spouse, annoying an employer, significant financial loss). Discretion about when to intervene with suggestions is essential and, for the most part, should be reserved for situations carrying potentially strong aversive consequences for the patient or others or extremely low probabilities of success. Also, the therapist should be careful not to jump in prematurely. The patient should be allowed the opportunity to identify potential problems via their own decision-making process.

Introduce activity scheduling early in treatment

Activity scheduling provides a convenient topic for beginning to model problem-solving strategies while at the same time increasing pleasurable activities to counter negative mood states. Most depressed patients are probably engaging in too few pleasurable or rewarding activities such as leisure and recreational activities, sporting events, and exercise. Most could benefit from increasing their pleasurable activities. A way in which this can be linked easily into the problem-solving process is to have as a problem 'Doing too few enjoyable activities'. A more detailed description of activity scheduling is provided in Chapter 5.

Focusing on activity scheduling begins to move the patient into a more action-orientated frame of mind, which is useful for problem-solving treatment. Activity scheduling provides a concrete topic for demonstrating the problem-solving treatment stages. In addition, activity scheduling offers a specific problem area on which the patient is almost guaranteed to be successful when they have difficulty identifying other problem areas.

Leave adequate time for problem-solving

Be careful not to spend too much time during the session either reviewing progress, discussing the patient's symptoms, or addressing other problems that come up between sessions. Therapists just beginning problem-solving treatment often run into serious time problems because of these factors. The review of progress should take no longer than a few minutes, and additional problems that come up in session, unless major in nature, can be agreed to be addressed at the start of the subsequent session. The bulk of time for the session should be used for goal setting, solution generation, and homework planning. Remember that a session should be a 'working session' and not an unfocused chat.

Stress the collaborative nature of treatment

Remember the axiom that the patient is usually the best judge of what their problems are and what they are able to do. The goal of problem-solving treatment is to teach the patient problem-solving skills, and to marshal the patient's existing resources into action in an organized and decisive manner. Therefore, the therapist should always ask which problem, goal, or solution the *patient* would like to pursue. Therapists should never assume or rush in with suggestions. The patient may not really want to follow through on the therapist's suggestions, but feel awkward about not doing as the therapist suggests. Remember, the *patient* is the expert on their own life.

It is not wrong, however, to throw in an idea for a possible solution or a way of framing an achievable goal if the patient has had the opportunity to fully explore this area themselves. However, such ideas should be provided tentatively and only as one idea amongst others.

Avoid direct advice

The therapist should usually avoid giving direct advice based on their own experience. An exception to this might be in providing information about educational or self-help resources, known about due to their professional activities. However, instead of offering even this general information, the therapist should consider using the problem-solving process to focus on how the patient will obtain the information on their own. The proper role for the therapist is as an expert in problem-solving, not as an 'advice giver'. The success of treatment rests upon the patient learning to competently apply problem-solving skills on their own, in the present and in the future, not upon advice provided for the moment by the therapist. Therefore, before offering a direct suggestion to the patient, first ask: 'What do you know about x? Do you know everything there is to know about x?' Most patients will readily admit that they cannot possibly know everything there is to know about just about anything, and this opens up the avenue for brainstorming about how to get further information on the topic. More than likely such a search will lead them to the information the therapist had in mind, but now the patient has the advantage of having learnt for themself how to access it.

The therapist may use certain specific treatment skills, as outlined in Chapter 5, if the patient wants to focus on symptoms of sleep and anxiety. To facilitate this, the therapist will provide limited information to guide the process.

The patient will often tempt the therapist to give advice and be more directive in therapy sessions, using such phrases as: 'I've no idea what to do', 'You're the therapist', 'I've tried everything', or 'I'm too tired to do anything'. Experience has shown, however, that if the therapist succumbs to the temptation of suggesting goals or solutions, the patient will either not implement the resulting plans or will counter suggestions with 'yes, but'. This generates fruitless discussion—time better spent in gently persuading the patient to identify their own ideas.

Balance aversive tasks with pleasurable activities

Many solutions to problems will require considerable effort on the part of the patient, and may require actions that will be uncomfortable to perform. When solutions require large amounts of effort, or are likely to be difficult (for example, breaking up with a boyfriend, talking with a boss about unsatisfactory work conditions, confronting a spouse about suspected infidelity), the therapist should work with the patient to counterbalance these events with some specific pleasurable activities. Although activity scheduling should be addressed in virtually all problem-solving treatments, in these particular circumstances a specific plan should be developed to offset a potential negative experience.

Disconnect other facts causing low mood from problem-solving successes

If the patient does not report improved mood after having successfully completed their homework, it is often due to outside events that have taken place, or a worsening of other existing problems. However, the patient may inaccurately attribute their low mood to failure of the problem-solving treatment. During the review of homework, try to identify possible other factors maintaining the low mood (for example, receiving bad news, having a physical illness) and disconnect them from the satisfaction of accomplishing the homework. In other words, the patient should not be allowed to assume that problem-solving treatment did not or cannot work to help them feel better. The other problems identified may then become future targets for problem-solving.

Keep discussion of symptoms and background brief

Remember that the symptoms of anxiety or depression are not the same as the problems for treatment. Therefore, prolonged discussion about uncomfortable symptoms (for example, tearfulness, guilt, poor sleep) only serves to distract from the focus of treatment, which is to solve the problems responsible for those symptoms. The therapist should keep the discussion of symptoms brief. Collecting background information such as age, marital status, and job is certainly reasonable, but the therapist should even keep this aspect of information gathering brief and in the spirit of 'getting to know you' versus a clinical interview. As the therapist works with the patient to develop the initial problem list, they are often surprised by how much symptom-related and psychosocial information they collect. Efficient use of time is a key aspect to problem-solving treatment, particularly in a primary care setting.

Allow silence

When working with the patient to generate goals, brainstorm solutions, and identify the steps to achieve the solutions, periods of silence should be allowed, to enable the patient to generate the necessary ideas. It is sometimes uncomfortable for the therapist, especially when first learning problem-solving treatment, to 'allow' silent blocks of time, without feeling a strong urge to jump in with their own ideas. However, as has already been noted, the therapist's ideas are usually not the best ones for the patient. Allowing silence provides the patient with the space to think things through, and also gives the unspoken message that they are to do the work in order for treatment to succeed. Therapists often find that once they have sat through some silences, the patient soon generates the ideas in a more organized and timely manner on future occasions. The patient is denied the opportunity to learn this skill when the therapist interrupts too soon.

Supervision

The supervised treatment of patients during training is an essential component of equipping therapists to be suitable problem-solving practitioners. Once trained, access to ongoing supervision is important. Supervision should be with an experienced therapist skilled in problem-solving treatment or a related cognitive behavioural therapy. Supervision may be individual, or it can just as usefully be undertaken in groups, with problem-solving therapists sharing ideas and solutions to difficult issues. Supervision enables the therapist to discuss with colleagues ideas about how to handle difficult issues which may come up in therapy. These issues may be related to the problem-solving process or be broader issues relating to, for example, risk or the patient/therapist relationship.

Avoid other therapy techniques

If the therapist has contracted for a brief treatment intervention (six sessions and, say, four hours' total treatment time), they will potentially lose the full impact of problem-solving treatment, as well as confuse the patient, if too many other techniques are introduced. One technique taught well can be more powerful and longer-lasting than several techniques given only brief attention. Problem-solving treatment is clearly not the only potentially effective psychological intervention for many patients, but it is one of the few shown to be of value within a brief intervention and, hence, the available time must be used appropriately.

Chapter 7

Three courses of problem-solving treatment

In this chapter, three worked-through examples of problem-solving treatment will be set out. These provide illustrations as to how problem-solving treatment unfolds over the six sessions. In the first example, of Elizabeth, a narrative history is provided alongside examples of problem-solving worksheets. In the examples of Jenny and Bill, the sessions are documented as they are written up after therapy with a brief history and then a focus on events and progress, as documented in the problem-solving worksheets. All three courses illustrate how problems and solutions change during therapy.

The case of Elizabeth

Elizabeth was a 43-year-old office administrator for a publishing company. She lived in a small village outside Edinburgh and commuted into the city each day to work. She had been married for 16 years. Unfortunately, her husband, who was seven years older than her, had severe arthritis which resulted in him being wheelchair-bound and unable to work. They had no children. Elizabeth was referred for problem-solving treatment following a nine-month history of worsening depression. Her main symptoms were low mood, tiredness, poor memory, and lack of concentration.

Session one

Elizabeth was still not completely convinced at the start of session one that her symptoms were due to a depressive disorder. Once a brief background history had been obtained, some time was spent at the beginning of this session explaining the nature of depressive illness and the physical and psychological symptoms that can occur. An explanation of problem-solving treatment was then given before

Box 7.1 Elizabeth's problems

1. Problems at work	Overworked—working 8 a.m.–7 p.m. Still doing work from old job. Being telephoned at home when not working. Previous attempts to resolve difficulties had failed.
2. Husband	Husband's illness. Although Elizabeth and her husband were spending a lot of time together, Elizabeth felt that her main role was as a nurse and that they were doing few 'normal' things which they could both enjoy.
3. Housework	Elizabeth felt that the house was becoming increasingly untidy and dirty and was in need of a spring clean, but she did not have the energy to do this. Already had a cleaner but she was not very effective.

a problem list was drawn up. Elizabeth's problems are set out in Box 7.1.

Elizabeth decided she wanted to focus on problem one in the first session, i.e. problems at work. She recognized that stresses of work were contributing to her symptoms, and thought they could possibly be improved. See Box 7.2. Firstly, Elizabeth decided that she needed a break from work in order to reassess the difficulties that she was facing. She set her first achievable goal as having two weeks off work. In brainstorming, the solutions she considered for having two weeks from work included taking annual leave, taking sick leave, and resigning from the job. She chose to take sick leave, and thought she should consult her GP to ask for a sick certificate. She already knew that her GP had advised her to have some time off work and decided that she should take his advice.

Box 7.2 Elizabeth's plan

◆ **Achievable goal**	Two weeks off work.
◆ **Chosen solution**	Would like a sick note from GP.
◆ **Implementation plan**	1. Ring work and inform them not coming in. 2. Ring for appointment with GP. 3. Explain to GP that not coping at work and needs time for treatment to work.

Elizabeth worked through the problem-solving techniques well. She had chosen from a potentially complex problem, namely her difficulties at work, a relatively straightforward achievable goal. This meant that she was able to quickly identify a solution that she thought would work and drew up a simple implementation plan to fulfil it.

The remainder of the session was spent doing activity scheduling. The implementation plan that Elizabeth had drawn up, whilst it may have been of potential help, needed strengthening in order for Elizabeth to have a sense of achievement. There was a danger that simply having time off work would be seen by Elizabeth as an admission of failure. The use of activity scheduling enabled her to identify other activities to be completed before the next session. It was particularly opportune that she was to have two weeks off in order to undertake these tasks.

The problem chosen for activity scheduling was not doing enough enjoyable activities, and the achievable goal was 'a treat a day'. Elizabeth chose the following activities to be undertaken during the subsequent week:

1. Going to the hairdressers.
2. Polishing her silver tea service.
3. Listening to classical music.
4. Arranging a shopping trip with her friend to Princes Street (in the centre of Edinburgh).

There was insufficient time in this first session to draw up a detailed implementation plan as to how these activities would be achieved. The therapist ensured that Elizabeth was aware that she would be most likely to achieve the homework tasks if she planned them in advance.

Session two (one week later)

Elizabeth had been successful in achieving her first goal, in that she had been to her GP who had, as she had expected, given her a sick certificate for two weeks. She had been partially successful with her activity scheduling. She had polished her silver tea service. This had given her significant satisfaction in that its unpolished state had been a source of irritation. She had also visited the hairdressers to have her hair done. She had not, however, gone shopping with her friend. There were two reasons for this. Firstly, she was worried that people from work might see her and think that she was 'skiving'. Secondly, when she had rung her friend, it had proved difficult to find a day that week for them to meet, and so she was arranging to meet up the following week. She had set herself one hour each day to listen to music whilst having a cup of tea.

Elizabeth described feeling a little better, although she was beginning to worry about work building up whilst she was away. She was also feeling guilty at having time off knowing the pressure that this would put upon her colleagues in the office.

Elizabeth was going to be off work for the whole of the second week before the third appointment. She wanted in this session to look at the problems at work and how she was going to deal with them. The worksheet for this problem is shown in Box 7.3.

Box 7.3 Elizabeth's problem-solving worksheet: session two

Problem

1. Working excessive hours.
2. Being telephoned at home when not working.

Achievable goals

1. To receive no telephone calls from work after 7 p.m.
2. To make an appointment to see her line manager in order to discuss how to reduce her workload.

Possible solutions

1. No out of hours' telephone calls.
   —Change telephone number and go ex-directory.
   —Not answer the telephone.
   —Have an answerphone.
   —Asking husband to answer the telephone and fend off unwanted calls.
   —Send a memo to all staff saying that she did not want to have any calls at home.
2. Making an appointment with line manager.
   —Write to line manager.
   —Telephone line manager.

Choice of solutions

1. Write a memo to work colleagues before going back.
2. Have husband answer the telephone in the evening and fend off unwanted calls.
3. Telephone and arrange an appointment with line manager for day of return to work.

Once Elizabeth had worked through the chosen problem and the two achievable goals successfully, there was time to review her activity scheduling plans for the coming week. Again, the importance of doing pleasurable activities was emphasized, in particular, the need to plan these and not to feel guilty about doing such tasks, which were integral to her recovery.

Session three (one week later)

Elizabeth was still in her fortnight's sick leave. Her mood had lifted noticeably since session one. She had telephoned work to arrange an appointment with her line manager for the day that she was returning to work. She had also done an e-mail to colleagues explaining that she did not wish to have out of hours' telephone calls and asking that she not be contacted out of office hours. She had not sent this directly but had sent it to her boss to have distributed as appropriate. Elizabeth had continued doing enjoyable activities. She indicated that she did feel better when having done something enjoyable. She had been to the cinema with her friend and had gone out walking with another friend.

In this third session, Elizabeth wanted to discuss what she was going to say to her boss at the forthcoming appointment. She also wanted to look at the difficulties she was having with her husband. She had approached her husband about answering the telephone in the evenings. He had expressed some surprise that she was unable to fend off calls herself but had readily agreed to take on this role once she had returned to work.

The question as to what Elizabeth would say to her boss was a continuation of the previous problem, namely working excessive hours, and could be viewed as setting out a more detailed implementation plan to solve this. Elizabeth was concerned that she might forget what she wanted to say and part of the session was spent in identifying the key messages she wished to convey to her boss. These included:

1. She was working excessive hours.
2. She was doing maternity cover for another colleague who was not expected to return to work and, hence, this extra workload was continuing for the foreseeable future.

3. She was often left to answer the telephones for other colleagues in the office when they went off on breaks.
4. She was still doing some work from her previous job in the company, which she had not felt able to hand over to her successor when she had been promoted.

Elizabeth decided that it would be helpful if she took a list of these concerns with her into the planned meeting.

The second part of the session was spent looking at the problems Elizabeth was having with her husband. She recognized readily that she could do little about her husband's (George's) illness. Indeed, she said that the fact of his arthritis was not a problem of itself. It was rather that because of all her other pressures, her contact with George was often spent assisting him with self-caring tasks and that they did little together that was enjoyable. These concerns were formulated on a problem-solving worksheet as set out in Box 7.4.

Box 7.4 Elizabeth's problem-solving worksheet: session three

Problem	Elizabeth feeling her main role was as a nurse and doing few enjoyable things with her husband.
Achievable goals	To do at least two planned enjoyable activities with husband in next week.
Possible solutions	To go to cinema. To take a holiday. To go out for a meal. To go for a drive to a local stately home.
Choice of solution	All of the above.
Implementation plan	Ring cinema to ask about disabled seating. Plan a holiday to Paris. Plan a day trip before returning to work. Arrange to cook an evening meal with George to discuss plans.

Session four (two weeks later)

Elizabeth had been very successful in planning sessions out with her husband, and had been to the cinema and had visited a local beauty spot. She was also planning a weekend trip to Paris for two months' time.

Elizabeth was now back at work and said that her colleagues had been very sympathetic. She had not yet met with her line manager who had had to reschedule the planned meeting. Having returned to work, she decided to set herself the goal of working only four days a week. She planned to discuss this with her manager at the meeting later that week. George had begun answering the telephone in the evening and had been successful in delaying calls until the next morning. However, Elizabeth was finding it difficult to cope with the anxiety of not knowing what the calls had been about.

Elizabeth's tasks for the coming fortnight were:

1. To continue weekly enjoyable activities with George.
2. To discuss with her manager, at the planned meeting, a possible four-day week and to stop all tasks from previous job.

Session five (two weeks later)

Elizabeth had met with her manager and agreed a plan to go to a four-day week. She saw this as a great achievement. She was planning not to work each Wednesday for a trial six-month period. It was agreed that she would not be telephoned on this day. She and her husband planned to use Wednesdays as an opportunity to go out together. Evening telephone calls had almost ceased, and Elizabeth had starting taking them herself, but agreed that if they became more frequent, she would get her husband to take them again.

Elizabeth picked up another problem from her problem list, which was housework. She believed that the house needed a spring clean. Elizabeth had been living in the house for the past two years. When she had moved into the house, she had 'inherited' the cleaner who had been employed by the previous owner. The cleaner was a well-meaning but somewhat elderly lady who, although reliable and honest, did not undertake the cleaning to Elizabeth's high standards. However, the cleaner had become something of a family friend and Elizabeth did not feel able to ask her to leave and employ another cleaner in her place. The problem, therefore, was how to get the house cleaned without upsetting her current cleaner.

The achievable goal was to arrange for the house to be spring cleaned by a contract cleaning agency. Elizabeth thought that this would be seen by her current cleaner as a major undertaking and something which she would not have been expected to do and, indeed, would probably welcome. Elizabeth undertook to ring two or three agencies that were advertising in the phone book and get quotes for them to undertake the work whilst she and her husband were having their trip to Paris.

Session six (three weeks later)

Session six consisted of a review of the progress which had been achieved so far, which was considerable. Unfortunately, the plan of reducing to a four-day week had not yet started. Difficulties had arisen with the employment of extra help both to cover Elizabeth's day off and also to cover some of the additional work that Elizabeth had kept on doing. Elizabeth, however, felt that her line manager was sympathetic to her difficulties and had agreed that she could take an extra two days' leave either side of the planned weekend to Paris. Elizabeth was unsure whether the goal of working four days a week would be ultimately achievable. She had arranged for a cleaning firm to spend two days in the house whilst she was in Paris. Her cleaning lady had not been upset by the plan. Elizabeth and George were doing one activity together each week.

There were no problems with termination. Elizabeth had fully understood the problem-solving concepts and was feeling notably better. The main potential difficulty she saw for the future was that work would become stressful and difficult again. However, the fact that the out of hours' telephone calls had been successfully managed meant that she did feel more able to cope with the workload during the day. She believed that the period off sick due to workload stress had affected, for the better, the pressure that was being placed upon her. She thought it was now more acceptable to say 'no' when she was asked to do additional work, as neither she nor her employers wanted her to get ill again.

The case of Jenny

The case example of Jenny is set out in the format used for recording the key elements of problem-solving treatment for use in supervision. The problem-solving sheets for each therapy session are included.

Jenny was more socially disadvantaged then Elizabeth, with fewer social or economic resources. However, she was still able to use the techniques of problem-solving to bring about worthwhile change. Jenny received six problem-solving sessions, described below.

Session one

Background

39-year-old divorced part-time cleaner in a nursing home. Lives in a rented house with two of her four children. Ex-husband (Dave) lives in same village and continues to visit (divorced 4 years ago). She is frightened of him; he occasionally assaults her and demands money.

Children

Rebecca (age 20)—one baby, lives 5 miles away; Jane (age 18)—at home; Shamus (age 15)—fostered, in trouble with police; Ben (age 9)—lives at home.

Work

Five mornings a week (cleaning) to top- up benefits. Enjoys work.

Social contacts

Has lived in village all her life but not seeing friends much because feeling fed up—'I'm no company'.

Clinical details

Describes being depressed 'for years' but worse over past seven months. Had been on amitriptyline 50 mg, stopped three months ago when took an overdose of 20 tablets.

Feels low, tearful, concentration poor, headaches, poor sleep(early morning waking at 3.00 a.m. and difficulty getting back off to sleep). Worries about Dave and money. Also feels guilty about Shamus being in care. Appetite increased, weight increased. Occasional thoughts of suicide, not serious, no plans.

Problem list

1. Money problems—£500 overdraft; husband not paying maintenance for Ben; wages too low.
2. Husband assaulting her when he visits Ben.
3. Overweight.
4. Shamus in care—'I can't handle him'.

Jenny chose her money problems as the focus for the first problem-solving session. Boxes 7.5 and 7.6 are the problem-solving worksheets for this first session.

Homework sheets

Tasks to be completed before next session:

1. List all outgoings.
2. Speak to Matron about more hours.
3. Visit notice boards at Post Offices and newsagents.

Box 7.5 Jenny's problem-solving sheet 1: session one

1. **What is the problem?**
   Income is less than outgoings.
2. **What are my goals?**
   To reduce outgoings to equal income.
3. **Solutions to achieve goals (as many as possible)**

	Pros	*Cons*
a) Stop buying cakes.	Also lose weight.	Difficult.
b) Buy cheaper cigarettes.	Need to cut down anyway.	Difficult.
c) List all outgoings.	Good.	It might depress me.

4. **Choice of solution**
   All three.
5. **Steps I need to take to achieve this solution**
   a) List all outgoings, with ways to reduce.
   b) Buy cakes only once a week.
   c) Change brand of cigarettes.

Box 7.6 Jenny's problem-solving sheet 2: session one

1. What is the problem?
Income less than outgoings.

2. What are my goals?
To increase income.

3. Solutions to achieve goals (as many as possible)

	Pros	*Cons*
a) Increase hours at work.	More hours at present job. Move to Fairlawns (another nursing home).	Not sure if more hours available. Don't like owners.
b) Go back on benefit.	? More money.	Take too long to come; not much more.
c) Look on notice board and in paper for new job.		
d) Advertise in village for new job.		
e) Get maintenance for Ben.	I should get £10 per week.	Tried already; Dave will be angry.

4. Choice of solution
a) Try to get more hours at current job.
b) Look for new/additional job on notice boards and in paper.

5. Steps I need to take to achieve this solution.
a) Speak to Matron about increasing hours.
b) Buy local paper—look in jobs section.
c) Look at Post Office notice board in three local villages.

4. Buy local paper.
5. Cakes, once a week only.
6. Cheaper cigarettes.

Session two (one week later)

Events

Big row with husband. She had mentioned maintenance. He had hit her in front of Ben and called her a 'slag'.

Progress

1. Outgoings all listed with budget plan—see Box 7.7.
2. Had spoken to Matron—no extra hours at present.
3. No jobs on notice boards.
4. One cake only.
5. Was using the cheaper cigarettes.

Problems for this session

1. Husband's assaults.
2. Leisure—not doing anything nice.

Jenny's worksheets for these two problems are shown in Boxes 7.8 and and 7.9.

Homework sheets

Tasks to be completed before next session:

1. See solicitor, Tuesday afternoon if possible, and discuss injunctions and maintenance.
2. See Smiths next week.
3. Ring Michelle for hair cut.
4. Carry on with electricity and gas economy.
5. One packet of cigarettes a day.
6. Write to electricity company—explain you will try to pay and want key meter.
7. Do a nice thing each day.

Box 7.7 **Jenny's outgoings and budget plan**

1. Electricity (£15 per week)—have key meter fitted; don't use tumble drier; cut down cooking; don't use fan heater.
2. Gas (£17 per week)—turn heating off.
3. Catalogue—pay off; no more purchases until Christmas.
4. Rent (£45 per week).
5. Telephone—Jane to pay for her calls; unplug and hide phone.
6. Buy food from supermarket, not corner shop.
7. Cut down on expensive food—no chops.
8. Cut down on alcohol (1/4 bottle martini day).
9. Cut down on cigarettes—40 down to 20 day; buy new brand with less tar.

Box 7.8 Jenny's problem-solving sheet 3: session two

1. **What is the problem?**
   No nice things happen to me.
2. **What are my goals?**
   To do a nice thing each day.
3. **Solutions to achieve goals (as many as possible)**

	Pros	*Cons*
a) Visit friends—Smiths.	Easy.	Will they be fed up.
b) Go to Bingo.	Enjoy.	Expense.
c) Go to pub.	Enjoy.	Drinking too much.
d) Brian (friend) come round.		Husband find out.
e) Have hair done.		Expense.

4. **Choice of solution**
   (a) and (e).
5. **Steps I need to take to achieve this solution**
   a) Contact Smiths and arrange to see.
   b) Ring Michelle for 'student cut'.

Box 7.9 Jenny's problem-solving sheet 4: session two

1. **What is the problem?**
   Husband hitting me.
2. **What are my goals?**
   a) Not to see him.
   b) Not to speak to him.
3. **Solutions to achieve goals (as many as possible)**

	Pros	*Cons*
a) Press charges of assault.	Punish him.	Frightened.
b) See solicitor re. injunction.		Expensive. Get tongue-tied.
c) If he tries to get in, call police.	Easy.	Won't come in time.
d) Access for Ben—Ben to wait outside or go to him.		Easy to say
e) If he rings up, refuse to speak.		

4. **Choice of solution**
   (b) Go to solicitor used in divorce; (c); (d) tell Ben he is going to have to wait for Dad outside.
5. **Steps I need to take to achieve this solution**
   Contact solicitor tomorrow.

Session three (one week later)

Events

No major scenes. Thinks she is feeling a bit better.

Progress

1. Couldn't make appointment with solicitor until next week.
2. Saw Smiths twice.
3. Has reduced cigarettes to 20 a day.
4. Electricity company will fit key meter.
5. Has had hair cut.

Problems

1. Still not enough money.
2. Need to see solicitor—assaults and maintenance.
3. Wants to stop drinking.

Jenny chose problem three as the focus for this session, her worksheet is shown in Box 7.10.

Box 7.10 Jenny's problem-solving sheet 5: session three

1. **What is the problem?**
   Drinking too much.
2. **What are my goals?**
   Stop drinking every day—instead, three times a week only.
3. **Solutions to achieve goals (as many as possible)**

	Pros	*Cons*
a) Stop altogether.	Cheap.	Difficult.
b) Drink only in company.	Less guilty.	Drink more in company.
c) Go to AA		Not an alcoholic.
d) Drink only in pub.	Would get me out.	Expensive.

4. **Choice of solution**
   Drink on alternate days—one bottle of wine over two days; visit pub twice—only have three martinis maximum.
5. **Steps I need to take to achieve this solution**
   Keep diary of how much I have drunk.

Homework sheets

Tasks to be completed before next session:

1. Continue with economy—electricity and gas; ration cakes to one Belgian bun; buy only one packet of 20 low tar cigarettes each day.
2. If husband tries to get into house—call police.
3. When Ben sees his dad—to wait outside the house.
4. Keep appointment with solicitor to discuss injunction.
5. List things that I used to enjoy and do one each day—gardening, puzzle book, aerobic video, music, reading magazine with cigarette.
6 Drink alcohol only on alternate days.

Session four (two weeks later)

Events

Bailiffs are coming next week to take goods because of mail order catalogue debts. Has been to Citizens Advice Bureau about debts and has decided she should stop work because she will have more money on benefit.

Progress

1. Has cut down cakes, cigarettes, and alcohol.
2. Solicitor's appointment not kept because of bailiffs.
3. Husband not coming into house—when he arrives, Ben is handed over on doorstep.

Problems

Leaving job—will miss work.
No new problem was discussed in this session, Jenny followed through plans from earlier sessions.

Homework sheets

1. Ring up solicitor on Friday to make another appointment. Taking back maiden name.
2. Speak to Matron re. going on benefits—leave nursing home on Friday.
3. Collect new benefit book from Post Office on Friday.

4. Look on notice board for cleaning jobs paying 'cash in hand'.
5. See Smiths or Webbs (other friends) once a week—only accept two drinks each time.
6. Saturday—buy 20 cigarettes; then cut down to 10 cigarettes a day.
7. Speak to friend in Bournemouth re. spending a week away.

Session five (three weeks later)

Events

Has given up job in nursing home—£20 per week better off and rent is paid. Bailiffs have taken television. Shamus (son) broke into house and threatened assault unless he was given money.

Progress

1. Has seen a solicitor—taking back maiden name; will get injunction.
2. Has left nursing home but got 2 hours a week cleaning in the village—cash in hand.
3. Drinking and cigarettes under control.
4. Will visit friend in Bournemouth in two months.

Problems

1. Son getting into house.
2. Overweight.

Jenny's worksheets for these two problems are shown in Boxes 7.11 and 7.12.

Box 7.11 Jenny's problem-solving sheet 6: session five

1. **What is the problem?**
   Too fat—11½ stone.
2. **What are my goals?**
   To reduce weight to 10 stone by October.
3. **Solutions to achieve goals (as many as possible)**

	Pros	*Cons*
a) Not to eat sweet things.		
b) Reduce alcohol—two glasses of wine on evening out.		

Box 7.11 Jenny's problem-solving sheet 6: session five *(continued)*

c) Exercise—bike, aerobics, walking.
d) Weigh myself once a week.
e) Attend Weight Watchers. Expensive.

4. Choice of solution
(a), (b), (c), and (d).

5. Steps I need to take to achieve this solution
a) Weigh myself each Sunday.
b) No sweets.
c) One exercise each day—walking, bike, or aerobics video.

Box 7.12 Jenny's problem-solving sheet 7: session five

1. What is the problem?
Shamus (son) will try to get in.

2. What are my goals?
Not to let him in.

3. Solutions to achieve goals (as many as possible)

	Pros	*Cons*
a) Keep door locked and windows shut.	Don't think he will smash window.	He will be upset.
b) If he gets in, phone the police.	Will stop him.	He may go to prison.
c) Telephone his foster family.		Embarrassed.
d) Let Social Services know.		Not usually any help.

4. Choice of solution
Lock doors and windows at night.

5. Steps I need to take to achieve this solution

Homework sheets

Tasks to be completed before next session:

1. Keep doors locked and windows shut at night to keep out son.
2. If son gets in, phone the police.
3. If husband rings up, don't speak to him.

4. Continue to look on notice board for another 'cash in hand' cleaning job. Put adverts in window in Post Office on Monday.
5. See Smiths or Webbs once a week—accept up to two drinks; plus see at lunchtime but no drink.
6. Daily exercise.

Session six (three weeks later)

Events

Feeling much better. Has had an interview for a full-time cleaning job in local pub/hotel.

Progress

1. Weight down (4lbs); cigarettes down (20 a day); alcohol down. Exercise 3 or 4 times a week.
2. Shamus has called again—not threatening; gave him £10.
3. No contact from husband (may have got solicitor's letter).
4. Hasn't put advert in shop.

Plans

1. Continue progress with weight, alcohol, and cigarettes.
2. Continue legal action against husband.
3. Find paid job.

Summary

In many ways, Jenny seemed beset by intractable problems which were not going to go away with a six-session course of problem-solving treatment. However, she worked through the problem-solving process and it helped her make important decisions about what to do:

1. Reduce alcohol and cigarettes.
2. See solicitor about ex-husband.
3. Clarify she was financially better off on benefits or in a full-time job.
4. Increase social activity and exercise.
5. Improved budgetting including getting a pre-paid electricity meter.

The problem-solving treatment did result in an improvement in Jenny's psychological symptoms, albeit many of her psychosocial problems remained.

The case of Bill

Background

31-year-old carpenter. Specialist in antique restoration. Made redundant 10 months ago. Married for 9 years. Wife, Lisa, works full-time as a life insurance saleswoman. Two children—Julie (age 5) and Daniel (age 2).

Bill and Lisa are having a lot of arguments. Lisa is working long hours and is often not at home. They cannot afford the mortgage payments on their house (bought three years ago) but cannot sell it because of low demand in the housing market.

Bill has been feeling 'down' for 4 months. Waking at 4 a.m.; feeling tired all the time; no interest in sex; difficulty concentrating; not enjoying life. Feels very guilty about not having a job and also for being irritable with the children.

No friends locally and is avoiding meeting his brother and mother with whom he usually has a good relationship. No previous history of depression.

Session one

Problem list

1. Not having a job, therefore, not enough money, no stimulation, no contacts outside the home.
2. No social contacts during the day.
3. Worries about being able to provide childcare for children.
4. Difficulties with wife, Lisa, whom he never sees.
5. House unsaleable.
6. House needs repairing and redecorating.
7. Mother has had major operation.

Bill chose problem two—social isolation—as the focus for the first problem-solving session, Bill's worksheet for this problem is shown in Box 7.13.

Box 7.13 **Bill's problem-solving sheet 1: session one**

1. **What is the problem?**
   Not seeing anyone all day except for the kids.
2. **What are my goals?**
   To get out of the house at least once a day.
3. **Solutions to achieve goals (as many as possible)**

	Pros	*Cons*
a) Join 'mother and toddler' group.	Friends for Daniel.	No men.
b) Go to job club (twice weekly group for unemployed)—social focus and skills acquisition.	Woman in charge a bit patronizing.	Childcare.
c) Visit neighbour who has kids.	Easy.	Shy.
d) Visit mum.	Be myself.	A burden/tire her.
e) Contact ex-workmate.	A good laugh.	Ashamed.
f) Go to playground with kids.	Easy.	No adults.

4. **Choice of solution(s)**
   a) Bill was aware that a local 'mother and toddler' group met twice a week in the church hall.
   b) Bill had spoken a few times with Sally, a neighbour, who had children of a similar age to Julie and Daniel.
   c) Bill's mum lived about five miles away.
   d) The children would enjoy this.
5. **Steps I need to take to achieve this solution**
   a) Ring mum and arrange to visit—will ring straight away.
   b) Will call on neighbour tomorrow to ask about toddler group and see if I can get invited in.
   c) Will at least go to park or to town once each day.

Session two (one week later)

Events

School holidays had started, so Bill was looking after both children all day—playing together well. Weather good.

Progress

1. Had visited neighbour and was going to toddler group next week. Not invited in, but spent 15 minutes chatting on doorstep.
2. Had visited mother at weekend with Julie. Lisa stayed behind with Daniel.
3. Had gone to the park each day.

Bill felt that he had made some progress. He had enjoyed going with the children to the park. Thought he had made some progress towards meeting people. Had enjoyed seeing mother and sensed she had enjoyed it as well.

Problem list

Relations with Lisa worse than ever—hardly talking. Can't go on. We don't talk we argue. Bill's worksheet for this problem is shown in Box 7.14.

Box 7.14 Bill's problem-solving sheet 2: session two

1. **What is the problem?**
   Lisa and I don't speak or we argue.
2. **What are my goals?**
   a) To speak to Lisa about how I feel and see if we can make things better.
   b) To arrange time with Lisa this week on our own, so we can talk.
3. **Solutions to achieve goals (as many as possible)**

	Pros	*Cons*
a) Go out for a meal.	Used to enjoy.	Expense.
b) Go out for a walk.	Cheap.	Who would look after kids? She doesn't enjoy walks—too tired.
c) Talk in the evening.		Both tired.

4. **Choice of solution**
   Get babysitter and do what Lisa would like for evening.
5. **Steps I need to take to achieve this solution**
   a) Ask sister-in-law (Mary) if she will have kids on Saturday.
   b) Suggest to Lisa this evening that they go out on Saturday.

Homework sheets

Tasks to be completed before next session:

1. Ring Mary for babysitting straight away.
2. Speak to Lisa this evening.
3. Go to toddler group on Wednesday.
4. Visit job centre (Bill still wanted to see if a job was possible).

Session three (one week later)

Events

Neighbour's husband has been round to warn Bill not to chat up his wife. Lisa very upset and accused Bill of wanting an affair.

Progress

1. Mary had agreed to babysit. In the event, Lisa said she didn't want to go out.
2. Had been to toddler group, had been made to feel welcome and thought would go again until argument with neighbour's husband.
3. No work at job centre.

Bill feeling very disheartened. Thought that the progress he had made in the first week had been undermined by events and that he was 'back at square one or worse'.

Problem list

1. Lisa coming home late most evenings (between 8 p.m. and 11 p.m.).
2. Need to sell house—can't afford it.

Bill's worksheets for these two problems are shown in Boxes 7.15 and 7.16.

Session four (two weeks later)

Events

Lisa has lost job 'out of the blue'. No idea how they will cope financially.

Box 7.15 Bill's problem-solving sheet 3: session three

1. **What is the problem?**
   Lisa coming home late most evenings (between 8 p.m. and 11 p.m.).
2. **What are my goals?**
   Lisa to come home and help put the kids to bed, and for us to have a meal together at least twice a week.
3. **Solutions to achieve goals (as many as possible)**

	Pros	*Cons*
a) Talk to Lisa.	Only solution.	Argument—'I work because we need the money'.
b) Talk to mum.	Always sympathetic.	Worry her; she doesn't really like Lisa.
c) Seek help (Relate).	We need outside help.	Lisa wouldn't go.

4. **Choice of solution**
   I will talk to Lisa and say this can't go on.
5. **Steps I need to take to achieve this solution**
   a) Choose time at the weekend to speak to Lisa.
   b) Ask how we can make it better.

Box 7.16 Bill's problem-solving sheet 4: session three

1. **What is the problem?**
   Can't afford the house.
2. **What are my goals?**
   Need to sell house.
3. **Solutions to achieve goals (as many as possible)**

	Pros	*Cons*
a) Finish decorating front room.	Looks a mess only half wallpapered.	No time. No interest.
b) Tidy garden.	Enjoy being outside in nice weather.	
c) Paint outside of house.	Looks a mess.	I can't do it myself and would cost money.

Box 7.16 Bill's problem-solving sheet 4: session three *(continued)*

d) Visit estate agent.	Need to sort out house first.

4. Choice of solution
(a) and (b).

5. Steps I need to take to achieve this solution

a) Finish wallpapering the front room (probably could finish it in a day if I stick to it)—ask Mary to have kids for the day.

b) Do gardening for two evenings when children are in bed.

c) Go to garden centre and buy some bedding plants.

Progress

1. Has finished decorating front room.
2. Lisa now at home—'she needs to see you'.
3. Garden looking more tidy.

Despite Lisa losing her job, Bill said he felt brighter. Worries about money offset by achievements and also the thought that he might be able to get a job, since Lisa could look after children.

Problem list

1. Need to get a job.
2. Need to sell house—house on market.
3. Lisa not coping.

Bill focused in this session on getting a job, his worksheet is shown in Box 7.17.

Box 7.17 Bill's problem-solving sheet 5: session four

1. What is the problem?
I need a job.

2. What are my goals?
To find work—anything will do, even if not in antique restoration.

Box 7.17 Bill's problem-solving sheet 5: session four *(continued)*

3. Solutions to achieve goals (as many as possible)

	Pros	*Cons*
a) Visit job centre again and ask for interview.	Best chance.	None.
b) Job section of local paper.	Usually jobs.	
c) Ask friends/brother.	May have contacts	Embarrassed.
d) Notice boards.		Poorly paid.

4. Choice of solution

(a), (b), (c), and (d).

5. Steps I need to take to achieve this solution

a) Visit job centre.

b) Ring a friend to see if he knows of any work.

c) Look on notice boards—newsagents, post office.

d) Buy local paper.

e) Finish decorating outside of house.

Session five (two weeks later)

Events

Lisa said that she had been having an affair with someone from work and she wants Bill to leave. He has been staying with his mum for a few days. He was very upset—'I didn't see this coming'. Had an appointment with a solicitor.

Session spent discussing the recent events. Bill was receiving support from family. He didn't want any further problem-solving at this stage.

Summary

This course of problem-solving was overtaken by events. At times, it had seemed that the problem-solving process was working. Bill had been able to identify clear specific problems and had made progress in sorting out solutions. He did not enjoy the role reversal—being at home whilst his wife worked. He had not appreciated that his wife had not always been truthful about the reason for her late nights.

Problem-solving treatment was not going to get Bill a job whilst his wife was earning more money than him and they were unable to afford alternative childcare. Similarly, problem-solving treatment was not going to sort out Bill and Lisa's marriage without a commitment on both sides.

Chapter 8

Potential problems with problem-solving treatment

Introduction

Although problem-solving treatment is a clear, organized, and structured treatment, the complexities of patients' lives mean that it is not always easy to conceptualize their difficulties as clear, defined problems. Even when clear defined problems are set, it is not always easy to formulate achievable goals. The skill of the problem-solving therapist is to facilitate the problem-solving process as best they can. It will of course be the case, however, that some patients' difficulties are too longstanding and entrenched to be helped by a six-session course of psychological treatment. The therapist needs to be aware of the limitations of problem-solving treatment and be realistic with the patient about the potential benefits that therapy can offer.

In this chapter, some of the common difficulties that arise during problem-solving treatment are set out. Case examples are given and suggestions put forward as to how the difficulties can be overcome. Potential problems with problem-solving treatment set out in this chapter are:

- No problems.
- Intractable problems.
- Problems with other people.
- Emotions as problems.
- Symptoms as problems.
- Poor engagement.
- Not done homework.

No problems

Some patients deny the existence of any problems in their lives. It may be the case that their lives are indeed problem-free and that the psychological symptoms they are experiencing have come out of the blue. However, this is very unusual for nearly all of us have problems, whether or not these problems are causing psychological distress. It is a rare and fortunate individual who has a problem-free life. Patients must be encouraged to identify their problems and not see them as a sign of weakness or failure. Patients should not worry as to whether the identified problems are really the cause of their symptoms.

If patients really cannot identify any problems, the therapist has two options—either to focus on a symptom as a problem (examples of how this might be done are given below) and/or to use one of the therapy techniques discussed in Chapter 5. In particular, even for patients with no problems, activity scheduling is likely to be an effective intervention. An example of a patient with no problems was Patricia (see Box 8.1 below).

Patricia denied that her life was anything other than very happy. She denied the existence of any problems. It was seemingly inexplicable to her why she had become depressed. Problem-solving treatment

Box 8.1 **Patricia**

30-year-old French graduate and trained teacher, married to a publisher, with an 18-month-old baby daughter. Stopped work after daughter was born. Several depressive symptoms for past three months.

- Happy marriage.
- Lovely daughter.
- Several friends.
- No wish to return to work.
- No money worries.

started with some activity scheduling. For Patricia, this first involved finding time for herself, to play the piano, which she had neglected since the birth of her daughter. Activity scheduling then looked at Patricia doing further enjoyable activities, both on her own and also with her husband and daughter. The first two problem-solving sessions, therefore, focused on activity scheduling. It was not until session three that Patricia burst into tears during the session and revealed to the therapist that she and her husband were having significant marital difficulties. These difficulties then provided the focus for the remainder of the treatment.

It became apparent during treatment that Patricia was a perfectionist in all aspects of her life. She had found it difficult, following her daughter's birth, to keep up the standards she set herself in the house, playing the piano, looking after her daughter, and being what she saw as a dutiful and loving wife. She was able to work successfully through some of these issues with her husband. Many of the problems were not dissimilar from the readjustments that all couples have to make following the birth of a child.

The importance of the story of Patricia is to emphasize the fact that patients do not necessarily reveal all their problems initially. It does take time for them to build up a trusting relationship with the therapist which enables them to talk more freely about difficulties that they face, particularly if these difficulties are of a personal and difficult nature. Even within the brief six-session structure of problem-solving treatment, patients do have time to build up an appropriate rapport with the therapist. The therapist need not feel concerned if key problems are not tackled immediately.

Intractable problems

Many patients present for a course of problem-solving with seemingly intractable and overwhelming problems. One of the important roles of the therapist is to avoid sharing the patient's hopelessness. The therapist needs to instil a sense of optimism that there are things which the patient can change. A good example of a patient with intractable problems is given in the vignette of Linda in Box 8.2 opposite.

Box 8.2 **Linda**

24-year-old single mother. Lives in second-floor maisonette with two boys—Rory (age 6), Kevin (age 4).

- Father has no contact.
- Mother lives one mile away but no contact since Linda divulged sexual abuse as a child from mother's ex-boyfriend.
- No job and no qualifications.
- No friends.
- Has felt depressed since Rory's birth.

Linda would appear on the face of it to have both longstanding emotional and social difficulties, with little in the way of personal or external resources. The challenge for the therapist here is not the eliciting of clear problems, but working with Linda to determine what she would like to change and then trying to find a way to assist Linda with this. Patients such as Linda do not expect 'miracles' from a course of therapy and, if given the opportunity, may well start to identify possible ways forward.

Linda identified two areas she wanted to focus on. Firstly, she wanted to re-establish contact with her mother. Secondly, she wanted a holiday for herself and the boys. During the course of treatment, Linda was helped to re-establish contact with her mother, planning what she was going to say and what was better left unsaid. By the end of the problem-solving treatment, Linda's mother was seeing the boys about once a week, which gave Linda a break from childcare. Linda did not speak to her mother about the child abuse issues. She considered seeking a course of therapy specifically to address this but decided that it was not an appropriate time for her to do this. The child protection issues about the abuse needed to be discussed. The details of the alleged perpetrator were passed onto the local Social Services Department for further action but the man's current whereabouts were not known. Linda was also helped to identify a means to go on holiday. She spoke to a social worker at the local family resource centre who helped her apply for a week's holiday with a charitable organization. By the end of therapy Linda had not heard whether this application had been successful, but she was feeling hopeful.

The example of Linda sets out the importance of identifying small changes which can be achieved by most, although not necessarily all, patients.

Problems with other people

Many problems people face in their everyday lives are linked to their relationships with others, whether family, friends, or work colleagues. Problem-solving treatment can help individuals tackle issues with others but, for there to be a resolution of the difficulties, often both parties need to be involved. Problem-solving can help the patient approach other people in a way which is likely to bring about a successful resolution. Patients can be helped to avoid exacerbating or worsening current difficulties.

Sometimes it is clear to the therapist that the patient is unlikely to be successful in bringing about a wished-for change with regard to the other person. A good example of this is the vignette of Paula in Box 8.3 below.

Box 8.3 Paula

Paula is 34 and works in publishing. She lives with her maternal grandmother. Paula's mother has severe alcohol dependence and Paula is very concerned she will die unless she accepts treatment. This seems realistic, as Paula's mother has had two hospital admissions with internal bleeding. Paula is often telephoned at work by her family because of her mother. She is seen as the 'strong person' to deal with the crises that her mother causes. Paula sees her parents most days.

Paula has longstanding anxious symptoms. She believes she will feel better if she persuades her mother to get help and stop drinking.

Paula's goal, set in the first treatment session, was to stop her mother drinking. The therapist felt pessimistic about the achievability of this goal, but Paula was adamant that it was the only goal that was relevant to her symptoms. Several solutions were looked at including:

- Taking her mother again to Alcoholics Anonymous.
- Going with her mother to the GP.
- Arranging for a private referral to a liver specialist.
- Speaking with her father to stop her mother having access to money to buy alcohol.

In the second treatment session, Paula reported that she had achieved some success. Paula's mother had agreed to see a liver specialist and had also agreed to attend AA. At the third session, Paula's mother was still drinking, but Paula remained hopeful that she could work with the family to stop her mother having access to money to buy more alcohol.

Paula arrived at the fourth treatment session very tearful because of an argument with her mother who had found out about Paula's attempts to stop her having access to money. Paula's mother had been very angry about this and told Paula to stop interfering with her life. The mother was now refusing to co-operate with any of the previously agreed plans. Paula did not feel that she had been supported by her family and now felt hopeless about the prospect of bringing about change. The therapist in the fourth session was able to refocus Paula's goals. A new goal was set—to stop being involved in the day-to-day crises concerning her mother. To this end, Paula looked at stopping her family ringing her at work, and she made the decision to move from her grandmother's house into a flat of her own. She limited her contact with her mother and father to a telephone call with her father once a week and visiting once a week.

The therapy with Paula is an illustration of how it is important for the therapist to allow the patient to focus on problems that they see as important, even if the therapist does not immediately see a way forward. It may well be the case that the patient has to fail in their first goals in order for more appropriate and realistic goals to be set and achieved.

Emotions as problems

Patients do not always identify clear practical problems as the areas they wish to work on. Sometimes the issues are concerned with emotions and symptoms. Two emotions that are often raised in problem-solving are anger and low self-esteem. These are difficult areas to work on within a problem-solving context and, if possible, the therapist should steer the patient towards more practical issues. However, on occasion, the issue of either anger or low self-esteem is the overwhelming factor for the patient and, if problem-solving is to be used as the therapeutic option, the therapist has to help the patient work through this within the format of problem-solving treatment.

An example of where the main identified problem was one of anger is illustrated in the clinical vignette of Karen in Box 8.4 below.

The therapist initially discussed with Karen that her anger was understandable in the context of what had happened. Karen felt that her sons had been emotionally damaged by having lived with her and her ex-partner, and it was understandable that she should feel angry about this. The therapist helped Karen clarify the nature and context of her anger, triggers for angry behaviour, and what might help when angry feelings emerged. Two goals were set:

1. To keep an anger diary looking at possible precipitants for anger.
2. To identify and use distraction options and record success in diary.

This process was of some value to Karen who was able to acknowledge that she did have some control over her anger and could manage

Box 8.4 **Karen**

Karen (age 38) is divorced. Two sons, aged 13 and 10. Following divorce had lived with female partner who was emotionally and physically abusive. After separation 18 months earlier was stalked and harassed by ex-partner who eventually went to prison. Karen often feels overwhelmed by angry feelings towards her ex-partner and hits out both verbally and physically. She just wants to stop feeling angry.

it. However, Karen wanted to stop herself feeling angry at all. In a later session, she set this as a goal. Brainstorming identified three possible options:

1. To write down all that had happened and burn the paper.
2. To talk with someone about what had happened.
3. To buy a doll and stick pins in it when she felt angry.

In the event, Karen decided to look at options one and two. She did write down some of what had happened but instead of burning what she had written, which she felt would be a cathartic experience, she shared it with her sister, who got angry in turn. Her sister's anger fuelled both Karen's sense of anger and also her guilt.

Alongside dealing with the anger, the therapist also worked on pleasurable activities for both Karen to do alone and with her boys. In identifying activities with her sons, Karen set up a pattern of fun activities which were enjoyable for all three of them. This helped assuage, in part, her guilt about what had happened.

Low self-esteem is a fairly common problem cited by patients in their problem list. It is a vague term and is not an ideal problem-solving focus. On occasion, however, patients will insist that this is the area of their lives that they do wish to work on in problem-solving and an example of this was Sharon, see Box 8.5 below.

Sharon was a very unhappy woman. The therapist started with the goal of working with Sharon to identify things that made her feel better. Sharon identified working, walking by the sea, and decorating her flat.

Box 8.5 **Sharon**

Sharon (age 42) is divorced from violent, controlling husband.

- Unable to see two sons unaccompanied (13 and 10) because of an incident three years earlier when she had hit son during an argument. Husband had called Social Services.
- Childhood in care; raped at 15.
- Lost job as care assistant because of incident with son.
- Wants to stop feeling useless.

Subsequent therapy treatment sessions focused on increasing Sharon's participation in these activities. In session three, Sharon set as a goal getting another job. This proved successful and she found a cleaning job.

One of the reasons that Sharon identified for her low self-esteem was the poor quality of contact with her sons. The contact she had always made Sharon feel worse because her ex-husband, or his family, had to be there when she saw the boys. Both they and the boys were often unkind to her. The therapist worked with Sharon to balance these visits, which Sharon felt it was important to continue, with an enjoyable activity. In this way, each visit with the boys did not lead to a worsening of her mood and self-esteem. Sharon did not want to look at possible options of seeing the boys without their father as her experience of the legal system and Social Services had left her feeling battered and disillusioned.

The example of Sharon is one in which the presence of intractable difficulties in a vulnerable individual means that the problem-solving process will have clear limitations. However, the alternative to problem-solving treatment for such patients is often that no intervention will be offered and no appropriate help received.

Symptoms as problems

The most common symptom which might be identified as a problem is sleep difficulty. Chapter 5 sets out how this can be handled as part of the problem-solving process. Sometimes lack of energy is identified as a problem. The patient needs to brainstorm possible solutions. A possible solution might involve setting a programme for exercise. A lack of exercise may be contributing to fatigue and, hence, lack of energy can be helped if patients take up physical activity. Aerobic exercise has been shown to be helpful for patients with depression in its own right and is thus a useful intervention.

Poor engagement

Some patients come to problem-solving treatment having been given little guidance as to what the treatment is. Although many of these patients, once the treatment has been explained, are happy to use the

Box 8.6 Jack

Jack is a 26-year-old unemployed man. He lives with his partner, a two-year-old son, and his partner's parents. He feels low and wants a 'place of his own'. He argues with his partner. His son is 'naughty'; does not sleep—'does my head in'. He is £2000 in debt.
Missed first appointment.
Second appointment—'I'm here for counselling'. Tasks:

1. Activity scheduling.
2. One child-focused activity.

Third appointment cancelled.

problem-solving process, there are others who do not engage in the process. An example of this is Jack, see Box 8.6.

Jack only attended one treatment session. He did not accept that part of feeling better was going to be dependent on him identifying goals and ways forward. Some patients in this situation continue to attend treatment sessions but do not do homework. They may be difficult to work with because of negative comments, both overt and passive. Jack voted with his feet and did not return.

Therapists need to remind themselves that the treatment does have to be collaborative and, unless engagement with the patient occurs, the treatment will not be successful.

Homework not done

There are many reasons why patients may not have done their homework tasks. This issue is discussed in detail in Chapter 4. Box 8.7 sets out a summary of the main reasons why this happens, together with the action necessary.

Box 8.7 Reasons for patient not doing homework

	Action
1. Patient unaware of need to do homework—'can't see the point' or 'I didn't know what I had to do'.	Explain treatment rationale and clarify plan.
2. Patient lacks motivation—'I couldn't face it' or 'there seemed no point' or 'too busy'.	Reinforce rationale and check goals/solutions manageable.
3. Patient unhappy with problem-solving treatment.	Open discussion with patient as to whether they want to continue.
4. Patient 'forgot'.	Explore reasons Explain rationale Check willingness to continue.
5. Patient felt 'pressurized'; not happy with tasks set.	Review problem and goals and emphasize patient choice.
6. Patient 'too depressed'.	Simplify tasks—do activity scheduling.

Chapter 9

Teaching problem-solving treatment

Introduction

This chapter sets out the structure of a two-day course to introduce problem-solving treatment to potential practitioners. The information in this chapter is based on courses which have been run for a range of professionals including GPs, nurses, medical students, and counsellors. The course does assume a knowledge of basic skills in delivering psychological treatments including confidentiality, time-keeping, and communication skills. The skills acquisition part of the course comprises five sessions, each of two hours' duration. Additional components can be added according to the context or more time can be spent rehearsing and practising the key skills.

In problem-solving training, emphasis is placed on the acquisition of skills rather than the acquisition of knowledge. Much use is made of role play in which the course participants practise being either the patient or the problem-solving therapist; their colleagues then provide feedback. This role play works best in groups of three or four. In groups of three, one participant practises being the patient; one, the therapist; and one, the observer to provide feedback. In groups of four, there are two observers. The individual role playing the patient may be given guidance as to the role or may use case vignettes from their own experience.

The observers need to be given guidance on how to provide effective feedback. Feedback should be structured according to positive points and areas for improvement, and observers should be specific about the behaviours commented on. Feedback needs to be as concrete as possible, picking out exactly what was said and what seemed helpful or unhelpful. If possible, alternative behaviours should be suggested as part of the feedback process.

The five key sessions teaching problem-solving skills are set out in this chapter. The structure of each session is described and examples of clinical vignettes are provided, together with handouts for course participants. Trainers will draw on the content of the earlier chapters of this book for the detailed information taught. Course organizers may want to introduce further sessions at the start or the end of training. At the start of training, information may be provided about the evidence supporting problem-solving (as set out in Chapter 2) and about the setting in which the problem-solving treatment is being delivered (for example, primary care, deliberate self-harm services). At the end of the course, further practical training in problem-solving can be provided (for example, videotaping the trainee therapists with simulated patients).

Session one: introducing problem-solving treatment and stage one

Aim

To introduce participants to problem-solving treatment, remind them of key communication skills, and provide the opportunity to practise stage one (explanation and rationale) of problem-solving treatment.

Objectives

By the end of this session, participants should be able to:

- Describe the seven stages and the structure of problem-solving treatment.
- Describe the goals of problem-solving treatment.
- Use key communication skills.
- Elicit symptoms and problems from a patient.
- Establish a link between symptoms and problems.
- Explain to a patient what problem-solving treatment is about.

Methods

1. Introduce the seven stages and goals of problem-solving treatment (slide presentation A—Appendix 1).

2. Demonstrate a brief (15-minute) problem-solving session using either role play between two trainers or a pre-prepared video.
3. Summary of key communication skills (slide presentation B—Appendix 1).
4. Introduction of stage one of problem-solving treatment—stage one handout (Fig. 9.1).
5. Stage one problem-solving treatment—theory and role play. Following the theoretical discussion of stage one, course participants then practise the technique in role play. Participants will need to divide into groups of three or four, with one taking the part of a patient, one the part of the therapist, and one or two watching and providing feedback. Role play in this early stage of problem-solving training is often helped by providing the participants with simple case vignettes, which set out ideas as to simple problems. Trainers should where possible use their own vignettes. Two appropriate examples (Annie and Adrian) are given below.
6. Opportunity for questions and clarification at the end of the session. Training session one should finish when all course participants have had the opportunity to role play stage one of problem-solving treatment. The session should end with an opportunity for questions.

Vignettes for role play

Annie

Annie is a 45-year-old hospital nurse, who lives alone. She is on sick leave because she can't cope with her work.

Symptoms

She feels low, tearful, and also has some difficulty falling asleep.

Background

She has never had a longstanding relationship and feels lonely. She finds her work difficult and is sometimes emotional. She is afraid to

Stage one

Making the link between symptoms and problems, and explaining the rationale of problem solving

Recognition of symptoms

The therapist starts with clarifying the reason(s) for appointment. Use an open question and listen actively to what the patient says.

'What brings you to see me today' or *'What took you to see your GP?'*

Summarize when necessary. React with empathy when required. Enquire specifically about the presence or absence of emotional symptoms using closed questions as necessary.

Recognition of problems

Once the therapist has recognized symptoms of psychological distress, establish the context in which these symptoms have developed. Seek to establish the patient's problems by asking questions such as:

'Are there any stressful things going on in your life at the moment?'
'I am wondering if there are any problems or difficulties in your life at the moment?'

More detailed enquiries about specific problems can be obtained by enquiring about potential problem areas such as:

1. Relationship with partner/spouse
2. Relationships with children, parents, siblings, and other family members
3. Relationships with friends
4. Work
5. Money
6. Housing
7. Health
8. Legal issues
9. Alcohol and drugs
10. Leisure activities

Making the link

Once the presence of both emotional symptoms and psychosocial problems has been established, a link should be made between the two. The patient should understand that symptoms are an emotional response to problems. The therapist then explains that problem-solving treatment will help the patient tackle their problems. Successful resolution of the problems will lead to resolution of the symptoms.

'The reason that you are feeling low and having headaches might be (is) because of the problems you are facing at work. If I can help you sort out those problems, I think your symptoms should improve.'

Fig. 9.1 Example of a training handout that summarizes stage one of problem-solving treatment.

make mistakes, and she can't talk to her superior about this. She also hates all the paperwork that comes with her job of co-ordinating a group of nurses.

Problem list

1. Problems at work:
   - Work is difficult and often stressful.
   - Afraid of making mistakes.
   - Dislikes paperwork.
   - Can't talk to superior.
2. Feels lonely.

Adrian

Adrian is 42 years old, married, with two children. He and his family moved to a new town about a year ago.

Symptoms

He is tired, feels down, and has back pain.

Background

The relationship with his wife is poor; he feels she constantly criticizes him. She is spending too much money and because of this the family has financial problems. Adrian and his wife never do anything nice together. He feels worried and stressed all the time.

Problem list

1. Relationship with wife:
   - Don't do anything nice together.
   - She spends too much money.
   - She is always criticizing him.
2. Financial problems:
   - Wife spends too much.
   - Not enough income.
3. Lack of pleasurable activities in new home town.

Session two: problem-solving treatment stages two and three

Aims

To introduce participants to the second (defining the problem to be worked on) and third (establishing achievable goals for problem resolution) stages of problem-solving treatment and to consolidate their skills in using stages two and three.

Objectives

By the end of this session participants will be able to:

- Help the patient clearly define a problem.
- State the problem in a clear and concrete form.
- Break down large problems into smaller and more manageable parts.
- Help the patient to set an achievable goal.

Methods

1. Introduction to stage two and three of problem-solving. The trainer should remind participants of the content of stages two and three of problem-solving using the handouts (Figs. 9.2 and 9.3). The patient handout on SMART goals should also be used (see p. 83).
2. Following the theoretical discussion about stages two and three, a case vignette can be used for defining problems and drawing up a problem list, and for the setting of achievable goals. The example of Gerti can be used (see Box 9.1). Initially, the clinical vignette of Gerti is shown to the whole group without the problem list. The participants then divide into pairs and draw up a problem list. Once this is done, there can be a group discussion about the problems and the example problem list is then shown. Participants then return to their pairs and choose one or more of the problems for the

setting of achievable goals. Once the participants have done this in their pairs, the trainer then goes round the class asking each pair for their achievable goals. There can then be a class discussion as to whether the goals chosen are SMART or not using the guidelines in the handout.

3. Role play stages two and three using vignettes from session one. Appendix 2 gives goals for the vignettes of Annie and Adrian.
4. Opportunity for questions and clarification at end of the session.

Stage two

Defining the problem to be worked on

Step 1: Defining the problem in a clear and concrete form

The patient should choose, in the first instance, one particular problem which is important to them and which the therapist and patient consider feasible for problem-solving treatment.

- Use clear unambiguous language.
- Specific behaviours if possible.

Step 2: Breaking down large problems into smaller and more manageable problems

- Clarify broad themes into specific issues
- Consider the following questions:-
  1. What is the problem?
  2. Why is it a problem?
  3. When does the problem occur?
  4. Where does the problem occur?
  5. Who is involved in the problem?

Sometimes patients will mention symptoms of their depression as problems they wish to address (for example, problems with sleep or energy). Although these symptoms are 'problematic', they are not objective life problems and, therefore, are not ideal for problem-solving.

Fig. 9.2 Example of a training handout that summarizes stage two of problem-solving treatment.

Stage three

Establishing achievable goals for problem resolution

Once the problem has been defined and clarified, the next stage is to choose one or more achievable goals. This involves establishing what, in particular, the patient would like to see changed about the problem. An emphasis should be placed on whether the goal can be reasonably achieved. It is important to take into account the balance between the patient's resources and obstacles.

As with the problem definition, emphasis should be placed on establishing a clear goal. However, the goal should not be stated in such detail that it generates a specific solution and prematurely aborts the solution generation process. This should be left for the next stage, during which the brainstorming of potential solutions takes place. Otherwise, the result is a poorly developed goal statement and a possible missed step.

Achievable goals are SMART goals:

Specific
Measurable
Achievable
Relevant
Timed

Good questions to ask in determining the patient's goals in relation to their problem are:

1. What do you want to do about it?
2. What do you want to change?
3. What do you want to be different?
4. What would make you feel better?

These questions enable the patient to move on from identifying the problem to clarifying what they wish to do about their difficulties. The patient will be taken through a process of clarification and definition:

Broad problem areas
⇓
Specific problems
⇓
Specific goals

Goals should be set that can be achieved, at least in part, before the next therapy session in order for patients to get a sense of achievement.

Fig. 9.3 Example of a training handout that summarizes stage three of problem-solving treatment.

Box 9.1 **Gerti**

Gerti is a 26-year-old shop assistant from Germany who married an air force serviceman (Scott) whilst he was stationed in Germany. She returned with him to the UK 18 months ago. Scott is now a salesman and they live in a rented two-room apartment. They have no children and no debts.

Gerti has a three-month history of feeling low. She has lost her sex drive and has put on 20 pounds in weight because of 'comfort eating'. She dislikes her job, but does not have the qualifications to get a better job. She dislikes their apartment and longs to own her own home.

She does not particularly miss Germany. Indeed, her family have visited twice and this was quite stressful. She and Scott are having worsening rows about her lack of interest in sex, his evening work which keeps him away from home three or four evenings a week, and her general dissatisfaction with life.

Problem list

1. Scott—arguments; no sex.
2. Work—dislikes.
3. Accommodation—wants to own her own home.
4. Weight gain.

Session three: problem-solving treatment stages four, five, and six

Aims

To introduce participants to the fourth (brainstorming), fifth (evaluating and choosing the solution), and sixth (implementing the preferred solution) stages of problem-solving treatment and consolidate their skills in using these stages.

Objectives

By the end of this session participants will be able to:

- Use brainstorming to identify potential solutions with patients.
- Manage the process of evaluating possible solutions and help the patient choose a preferred solution.
- Draw up implementation plans for chosen solutions.

Methods

1. Introduce the theoretical background to stages four, five, and six. Use handouts (Figs. 9.4–9.6).

Stage four

Brainstorming

Once an achievable goal has been set, the patient is asked to generate a range of potential solutions. Teaching individuals to think creatively of a range of possible solutions is based on the premise that the availability of a number of alternative actions will increase the chances of eventually identifying particularly effective solutions. In other words, the 'first idea' that comes to mind is not always the 'best idea'.

It should be emphasized to the patient that they should try to generate as many solutions as possible via 'brainstorming' techniques. Potential solutions should not be discarded or prejudged, even if initially they seem to be silly or unworkable. Teaching patients to think of multiple solutions helps them to become more flexible in their perspective on problem resolution.

- The quantity of solutions generated is important. The greater the number of potential solutions, the greater the chances for successful resolution of the problem.
- The patient should feel free to combine ideas and modify them as they develop.
- The patient should not judge the ideas until the brainstorming process is completed.
- If the patient is having great difficulty developing solutions, they should be encouraged to think how other people might respond to the problem, or to deliberately invent a solution that is blatantly silly.
- In order to facilitate brainstorming it is helpful for the therapist professional to make statements such as 'what else can you think of?', 'think freely', 'be playful with your ideas', 'don't prejudge', and 'throw caution to the wind'. Therapists should steer away from statements such as 'can you think of anything else?' and 'can you think of any other ideas?' as these invite the response 'no'.
- Consider the 'brick technique'.

Fig. 9.4 Example of a training handout that summarizes stage four of problem-solving treatment.

Stage five

Evaluating and choosing the solution

Once a range of possible solutions has been identified, the therapist teaches the patient to evaluate the alternative solutions by implementing decision-making guidelines. Specifically, the patient is asked to consider the 'pros' and 'cons' for each potential solution. Effective solutions are those that not only solve the problem but also minimize negative outcomes for the self and others. As with facilitating brainstorming, it is helpful to frame comments in an open-ended fashion, such as 'what are the advantages and disadvantages of . . . ?', which implies that there are necessarily some of each dimension.

The patient should be encouraged to consider whether each potential solution will:

1. Make a significant impact on the problem.
2. Have advantages or disadvantages in relation to the patient's time, effort, money, or emotional distress.
3. Have positive or negative effects on the patient's friends and family.
4. Have the likelihood that they can carry it out in a satisfactory fashion.

As with all the problem-solving stages, it is ideal for the *patient* to evaluate his or her own solutions. However, there are two occasions in which it is acceptable for the therapist to introduce information. The first is when the patient is overlooking a negative consequence, either for themselves or others, which is extreme. The second instance is when the patient mentioned an advantage or disadvantage earlier during the session, such as during the brainstorming phase, but appears to have forgotten this in the current stage.

Once the pros and cons have been considered for each potential solution, the patient selects a preferred solution or solutions. Ideally, the solution selected should achieve the stated goals while carrying the least personal and interpersonal disadvantages connected with it. Consider:

- How feasible is the solution?
- Will the solution have an impact on the problem?
- More than one solution may be chosen.

Fig. 9.5 Example of a training handout that summarizes stage five of problem-solving treatment.

2. Role play stages four, five, and six, using previous vignettes. Appendix 2 contains additional information about Annie and Adrian. Course participants can use vignettes from their own practice.
3. Opportunity for questions and clarification at the end of the session.

Stage six

Implementing the preferred solution(s)

Once chosen, the steps required to achieve the solution are identified and planned. Detailed actions and specific dates, times, etc. should be determined. This step helps to ensure that 'good intentions' are translated into definite action. The therapist should ask:

- 'What needs to be done or obtained?'
- 'Where is it to be done?'
- 'Whom does it involve?'
- 'How will it be done?'

The patient must identify and choose tasks that they feel comfortable implementing, but the therapist should ensure that the tasks are sufficient to satisfy the requirements of the solution as well. Sometimes this means that the solution may need to be broken down into more simple sub-steps.

- Consider role play
- If patient worried about a task, be specific about detail
- Patient must be clear about homework tasks
- Tasks should be written down
- The therapist must ensure that implementation plans are sufficiently challenging for the patient to get a sense of achievement on successful completion but not overwhelming or daunting

Fig. 9.6 Example of a training handout that summarizes stage six of problem-solving treatment.

Session four: problem-solving stage seven and role play in all seven stages

Aim

To introduce participants to the seventh stage of problem-solving treatment and consolidate their skills in delivering all seven stages of problem-solving treatment.

Objectives

By the end of this session participants will be able to:

- Manage the evaluation of progress—stage seven.
- Role play all seven stages of problem-solving treatment.
- Embark on subsequent problem-solving sessions.

Stage seven

Evaluation and next steps

In stage seven, the evaluation phase, the therapist should ask the patient about their success with the homework and praise any progress. The therapist can then discuss problems and difficulties, bearing in mind that patients may selectively attend to failures. It is important to praise all successes, however small, without being patronizing.

The review of progress should be followed by asking about the impact of the success on the patient's symptoms. This reinforces the explanation of the problem-solving process and its rationale.

In discussing failures, the therapist should communicate that they see the patient's potential for effective coping as this facilitates a positive problem-solving approach. If difficulties have arisen, the reasons should be examined:

- Should the goals be defined more clearly?
- Are the goals realistic?
- Have new obstacles arisen?
- Are the implementation steps difficult to achieve? If so, why?
- Is the patient truly committed to working on the problem?

The answers to these questions will guide this session. If the problem is simply too difficult to tackle (usually due to the patient not having sufficient control over the source of the problem), then it is reasonable to go onto another problem or to modify the goal to focus on aspects of the problem over which the patient has more control.

If the patient has not completed the homework tasks, they may not have understood the central role of homework. It should be emphasized that progress occurring between treatment sessions is more important that progress achieved within a session. The therapist should stress that the goals and solutions were chosen by the patient, not by the therapist.

If the patient has successfully completed the homework tasks, then a new problem may be chosen and discussed using the problem-solving process.

Fig. 9.7 Example of a training handout that summarizes stage seven of problem-solving treatment.

Method

1. Explanation and discussion of problem-solving treatment stage seven. Use handout (Fig. 9.7).
2. Role play stage seven using either previous vignettes or vignettes devised by themselves.
3. Role play all seven stages of problem-solving treatment. The course participants will have had the opportunity to practise in detail the individual stages of problem-solving treatment. The next stage is

to consolidate this by role playing a fresh vignette going through from stages one to seven. This is often best done if participants bring their own vignettes to the training which makes it easier for them to stay in role. It needs to be emphasized that reasonably simple case vignettes should be chosen and that the participants role playing the patient do not make the role play unduly difficult—this is for early training after all! The role play can be undertaken in the usual way with one participant role playing the patient, one role playing the therapist, and one or more acting as observers, providing feedback.

A useful technique, if resources are available, is to videotape this role play. Participants are informed that the problem-solving stages need to be completed within a 20-minute session in order for the videotapes not to be overly lengthy. All participants need to role play a patient and a therapist.

Feedback occurs in small groups in which the videotapes are observed by the role play participants. It is important to handle the feedback sessions carefully using the feedback guidelines noted on page 163. The groups for feedback should not be more than five or six in order that everyone feels comfortable both about providing and receiving feedback. There are several advantages to using videotapes of role play for training. Not only can participants see themselves and provide their own personal feedback on the role play, but also there is the opportunity to rewind and repeat certain segments of the recording and consider what would be alternative ways of responding to the therapy content of the role play. In addition course participants can provide initial feedback which helps them identify good and less good problem-solving techniques. If role plays are to be recorded, the organizers of the training need to ensure that there is sufficient time for all participants both to undertake a role play and to receive feedback. This is likely to take another whole training session.

4. Opportunity for questions and clarification at the end of the session.

Session five: potential problems with problem-solving treatment and how problem-solving develops over six sessions

Aim

To consolidate knowledge of problem-solving treatment by discussion of potential problems which might arise during problem-solving treatment. To prepare for the full course of problem-solving.

Objectives

- To elicit participants' own concerns about problem-solving treatment.
- To identify common areas of difficulty with problem-solving treatment.
- To discuss how problem-solving treatment fits in within six sessions.
- To discuss activity scheduling, if not already raised.

Method

1. Brainstorm with the group, potential difficulties that they have identified with problem-solving treatment. These difficulties should be written up on a board or a sheet and referred to throughout the session in order to make sure that all the points are covered. Once the group have identified possible problems, there can then be a discussion as to how these might be overcome or how realistic the concerns are. Although this discussion should be led by the course trainers, useful and helpful comments often come from other members of the group.
2. Identify potential problems with problem-solving treatment and reinforce elements needed for effective problem-solving. The trainers should draw relevant examples from Chapters 5 and 8. The precise examples will depend on how previous discussions have gone. Trainers may bring in new material and emphasize points already discussed.

3. Run through one or more case vignettes of a course of problem-solving, using examples from Chapter 7. The use of these examples illustrates how problem-solving treatment develops over the six sessions. Trainers should reinforce the following points:
   - Patients take more of a lead in the problem-solving process as sessions develop.
   - Summarize progress and successes, remembering what has already been achieved can help if there are current set backs.
   - More work is done outside sessions as treatment progresses.
   - In the final sessions(s), leave time to consider what future problems may be worrying the patient.
4. Discuss role of activity scheduling using the patient handout on page 101.
5. Opportunity for questions and clarification at the end of the session.

Ongoing training and supervision

The training in problem-solving treatment as outlined in this chapter does not equip individuals to undertake problem-solving treatment without gaining supervised training experience with patients. In the problem-solving studies outlined in Chapter 2, trainee therapists treated a minimum of five patients, under supervision, before being equipped to deliver the problem-solving treatment.

Supervision should be provided by an experienced problem-solving or cognitive behaviour therapist. It is often helpful for supervision to be provided in groups of two or three in order that participants might learn from one another as well as from the supervisor. Supervision should occur, as a minimum, on three occasions with each patient during training—once after the first therapy session, once during the treatment sessions, and once following the end of treatment to discuss how the course of treatment went. Supervision at its best includes videotaped or audiotaped sessions in which the supervisee identifies areas of the therapy session which they wish to discuss with the supervisor and their fellow supervisees in order to learn from their feedback.

Appendix 1

Teaching aids

Session one, slides A: Introduction to problem-solving treatment

1

SEVEN STAGES OF PROBLEM-SOLVING TREATMENT and GOALS OF PROBLEM-SOLVING

2

Seven stages

1 EXPLANATION AND RATIONALE
2 PROBLEM DEFINITION
3 ESTABLISHING ACHIEVABLE GOALS
4 GENERATING SOLUTIONS
5 EVALUATION AND CHOICE OF SOLUTION
6 IMPLEMENTATION
7 EVALUATION

3

Rationale

EMOTIONAL SYMPTOMS	*PHYSICAL SYMPTOMS*
◆ Low mood	◆ Sleep disturbance
◆ Loss of enjoyment	◆ Appetite change
◆ Worries	◆ Tiredness
◆ Poor concentration	◆ Headaches
◆ Irritability	◆ Aches and pains
◆ Hopelessness	

4

Problem list

- Relationship . . . . . partner/spouse
- Relationships . . . . children/other relatives
- Relationships . . . . friends
- Work
- Money
- Housing
- Health
- Alcohol and drugs
- Legal issues
- Leisure activities

5

Linking together

- Problems cause symptoms
- If problems can be resolved, symptoms will improve
- Problems can be resolved using problem-solving

6

Definition and breakdown of problem

- State the problem in a clear concrete way
- Control
- Feasibility
- Very clear definition

7

Breaking the problem down

- Helps with clearer definition
- Enables sense of control and achievement earlier
- Fact or assumption?
- What, when, where, who, and how?
- Impact on their life

8

Establish achievable goals

- What would they like to see changed?
- Can it be reasonably achieved?
- Resources v. obstacles
- Short-term at the start
- Medium-term over time
- Long-term later
- Clarity without rigidity

9

Achievable (SMART) Goals

- **S**PECIFIC
- **M**EASURABLE
- **A**CHIEVABLE
- **R**ELEVANT
- **T**IMED

10

Generating solutions

- 'Brainstorming'
- The more, the merrier
- Mix and combine
- Avoid judgement
- PRAISE ++++

11

Choosing a solution

- Pros and cons
- Effect on family, friends, and colleagues
- Actual impact on problem
- Ability to carry it out
- Avoid therapist choice unless negative impact
- More than one is OK

12

Implementing preferred solution

- Detailed, planned steps
- Minimize chance of inaction
  —Rehearse interview/confrontation
  —Go back if necessary
  —Be specific about time, frequency, difficulties
  —Write it down

13

Evaluating the outcome
(Follow-up sessions)

- Review homework
- Recognize any steps and PRAISE
- Link task completion to symptom reduction
- Review difficulties

14

Potential difficulties

- Was the goal clearly defined?
- Was the goal realistic?
- Have new obstacles arisen?
- Are the implementation steps too hard?
  —What else could they do?
- Are they committed to working on the problem?

15

Moving on

- Return to problem list
- Follow the same process
- Stay positive
- Consider activity scheduling

16

Activity scheduling

Most people will benefit; always suggest if:

1. Lack of pleasurable events identified on problem list
2. Other problems are outside person's control
3. When solution is likely to have a negative outcome in short term
4. When person insists that they have no problem

17

Summary

- PST is a brief psychological treatment
- It is collaborative and positive
- It follows specific steps
- It increases a person's sense of control over their lives
- It involves the person working outside the session
- IT WORKS!!

Session one, slides B: Review of communication skills

1

Brief rehearsal of communication skills

2

Questioning

- Open questions
- Probing questions
- Prompts
- Closed questions
- Leading questions
- Overlapping questions

3

Listening and responding

- *Active listening*
  —Clarifying now and then
  —Repeating in your own words
  —Reacting with empathy
- *Summarizing*
  —Check out what has been said

4

Listening and responding

- *Explaining*
  —Adjust to individual patient
  —Follow patient's pace
  —Assess understanding
- *Negotiating*
  —Therapist guides, patients chooses
  —Seek plan both happy with

5

Non-verbal communication

- *Therapist*
  —Make eye contact
  —Try to have a relaxed posture
  —Inviting gestures are sometimes helpful
- *Patient*
  —Expression on face tells about emotion
  —So does his or her posture
  —So do gestures

Appendix 2

Additional information for case vignettes used in training

Annie

Problem 1: work

Annie's goals were:

(a) Look at ways of reducing stress at work.

(b) Find a way to increase confidence in work.

(c) Sort out way of making paperwork less of a burden.

Brainstorming solutions for goal (a)

	Pros	Cons
1. Find out if there are courses which might help increase skills.	I might even enjoy a course.	Lack of time; difficult to find.
2. Discuss alternative ways of doing work with a colleague.	Might come up with new ideas.	I only have one colleague and her work is quite different.
3. Talk with job supervisor about stress.	She might have a good suggestion.	Difficult—I have difficulty communicating with her; she might make a fool of me.
4. Start looking for another job.	Saves a lot of stress if I can find it.	Might be difficult finding it; feel like giving in too quickly.

Annie's choice of solution was a combination of 3 and 4.

Plan

1. Make an appointment with job supervisor tomorrow for some time this or next week. If she is not available tomorrow, find out when she will be and make sure to make the appointment this week.
2. Start looking on the internet and in newspaper today for some ideas about what I might like to do. Call job centre tomorrow. Make a list of available jobs.

She gave goal (a) priority and did not follow through with (b) and (c) because she did not feel they were as relevant.

Outcome

She arranged a meeting with the job supervisor and discussed the problem. This went better than expected. Together they made a plan to look at the availability of other jobs in the hospital for which she was qualified. It turned out that there were a few options. She applied for them and after three months started in another job (where she still enjoys working a year later).

Problem 2: feeling lonely

SMART goal

Plan at least two leisure activities a week—one to do alone, one to do with other people.

Brainstorm solutions

	Pros	Cons
1. Go shopping.	Like shopping.	Might spend too much.
2. See a film.	Like going to movies.	Friend might not be free.
3. Go for a swim.	Relaxing.	An effort.
4. Visit a friend.	Nice.	I might intrude.
5. Play music.	Like it.	
6. Rent a nice video.	Like movies.	Might feel lonely.

Choice of solution(s)

1. Rent a video and listen to music at home at least once or twice a week.
2. Go for a swim or shopping with a friend at least once a week.

Plan

1. Call my friend tonight and ask her if she wants to join me shopping and set a date. Suggest that we go for lunch together as well. If she is not home tonight, then call again tomorrow, until date is set. If she wants to but cannot come this week, then set date for next week and call another friend to see if she might want to go this week. Make the plan sound good!
2. Find out opening hours of local swimming pool before I call friends.
3. Go to the video shop on Wednesday and choose a nice video. Make sure I create a cosy atmosphere; unplug phone.

Outcome

First friend was very surprised by initiative. They went shopping together and more or less arranged to do this and other things on a regular basis at least once a fortnight.

Another friend whom she called was more busy and she did not succeed there. She remembered that her sister-in-law (brother's wife) enjoyed swimming and had had plans to go for some time. She called her. They went for a swim and do so almost every week, which they both enjoy.

Listening to music does not work—she starts 'thinking' too much; it does not relax her enough. Watching a video does help—it is more distracting. She made a list of videos she might want to see in coming weeks.

Adrian

Problem 1: relationship with wife

Goals

(a) Plan at least one pleasurable activity per week together.

(b) Discuss with her our financial situation and make new/alternative agreements about our family expenditure.

(c) Find a way to express my feelings to her about her criticisms.

Brainstorming solutions for goal (a)

	Pros	Cons
1. Go to gym together.	Each on own level, but still together.	Might be too individual; too out of breath to talk.
2. See a movie together.	Both like movies; out of house together.	Cannot talk.
3. Go out for a meal.	Both enjoy nice meals.	Too expensive.
4. Play games with children together.	Nice; kids will be thrilled because it is unusual.	
5. Go cycling together with kids.	Nice and active; kids will love it.	Difficult to plan.

Choice of solution(s)

1 and 4.

Plan

1. Talk gym plan over with wife at weekend and set a date; phone gym about opening hours and costs; make an appointment.
2. Talk with wife tonight or tomorrow, agree on a time when children are back home from school; plan what we will do together; arrange follow-up immediately if it is nice.

Outcome

Talked with wife; they made an achievable plan for the same week. They did a number of activities with the children and it was fun. Planned with children to do this on regular basis. Talked with wife about gym plan. She agreed; have not been yet. Adrian continued to work on this problem during treatment and thought it had really helped.

Problem 2: financial difficulties

Due to:

(a) Overspending (by my wife).

(b) Lack of sufficient income.

Goals

Goal a: discuss with wife financial situation and make new/alternative agreements about our family expenditure
Goal b: make a plan to increase income

Brainstorming goal (a)

	Pros	**Cons**
1. Make a list of incoming money.	Easy; clear.	
2. Make a list of my and her expenditure.	Clear.	She will not believe it.
3. Discuss list with wife.	Necessary; might help.	Difficult; she might not want to.
4. Seek expert advice (Citizens Advice Bureau).	Makes it easier for me.	She will not want to involve someone else.
5. Early in month, place an amount of money out of her reach.	Leaves money at the end of the month.	Wife will be very angry.
6. Buy necessities before she can get she hold of the money.	At least priorities are taken care of.	Will only work once; will be very angry.

Choice of solution(s)

1, 2, and 3 first; possibly 4.

Plan

1. Start making list of income and expenditure when she is out tomorrow. Go on working on it this week and make sure I finish

by Friday. If I can't manage Friday, Monday at the latest. Use bank copies and be very concrete.

2. Tell my wife, when I have completed my list, that I want to discuss our financial situation as soon as possible and set a date and time with her; make sure that she does not put it off. Then show her the lists. Ask her for suggestions on how we can cut down on expenditure. Discuss my own suggestions. If it does not work, suggest asking advice.

Brainstorming solutions for goal (b)

	Pros	Cons
1. Look for a different job.	Might enjoy a change.	Difficult to find.
2. Find an additional job.		No time; I can't do any more.
3. Ask wife to start working.	Would really help; she might enjoy it; she would spend less because less time.	She might not want to.

Choice of solution(s)

1 and 3.

Plan

Start looking for ads in newspaper and internet tomorrow; make a list and start phoning a few every day. While I am working on this, also talk with my wife, at the weekend, after the kids are in bed. Tell her about my actions and ask her how she feels about going back to work now the kids are at school. Think through how to raise the subject in a positive way, pointing at the advantages for all of us of having a bit more of a margin each month, and what we could do with it.

Outcome

Made a list; not many jobs available.

Told wife he wanted to talk their financial situation over at the weekend and she agreed, reluctantly. Reacted positively to his suggestion that he find an additional job. She was surprised with his suggestion that she started working as well and raised some problems about what to do about childcare. She agreed she would start looking to see if there was any work available for her. Any decisions would be agreed jointly. Adrian decided he knew now what steps to take and it was no longer necessary to do this with a therapist.

Problem 3: lack of pleasurable activities in new home town

Goal

Increase number of pleasurable activities

SMART goal

Plan a pleasurable activity at least once a week, etc.

Brainstorming

	Pros	Cons
1. Go to library for information.	Easy.	Don't expect much.
2. Enquire at local community center.	Easy; around the corner.	Probably no activities I like.
3. Look for leisure activities in phone book.	Easy.	
4. Ask a neighbour for suggestions.	Might have good suggestions; perhaps do something together?	I might seem foolish.
5. Surf the internet.	Easy; might give bunch of new ideas.	Probably not locally.

Choice of solution(s)

2, 4, and 5.

Plan

1. Go to community centre tomorrow.
2. Friday, when I know my neighbour is at home early, pop in with one of the kids and ask for advice and suggestions.

3. Surf the internet today or if I don't manage today, then tomorrow, and look for nice things like a theatre group, etc. Call immediately or the day after if I find any phone numbers.

Outcome

Idea 4 went well. Neighbour had lots of suggestions. One was jogging together. They agreed they would both like that and arranged a time. They do this regularly now. Community centre did not have much. Still working on other options, but is quite happy with this first step and decided it was enough for him.

References

Alexopolous GS, Raue P, Arean P (2003). Problem-solving therapy versus supportive therapy in geriatric major depression with executive dysfunction. *American Journal of Geriatric Psychiatry* **11**; 46–52.

Arean PA, Perri MG, Nezu AM, Schein RL, Christopher F, Joseph TX (1993). Comparative effectiveness of social problem solving therapy and reminiscence therapy as treatments for depression in older adults. *Journal of Consulting and Clinical Psychology* **61**; 1003–10.

Barrett JE, Barrett JA, Oxman TE, Gerber PD (1988). The prevalence of psychiatric disorders in a primary care practice. *Archives of General Psychiatry* **45**; 1100–1106.

Barrett JE, Williams JW, Oxman TE, Frank E, Katon W, Sullivan M, *et al.* (2001). Treatment of dysthymia and major depression in primary care: a randomised trial in patients aged 18–65. *The Journal of Family Practice* **50**; 405–412.

Beck AT, Ward CH, Mendelson M (1961). An inventory for measuring depression. *Archives of General Psychiatry* **4**; 561–571.

Billings AG, Moos RH (1981). The role of coping responses and social resources in attenuating the stress of life events. *Journal of Behavioural Medicine* **4**; 139–157.

Catalan J, Gath D, Edmonds D, Ennis J (1984). The effects of non-prescribing of anxiolytics in general practice. *British Journal of Psychiatry* **144**; 593–602.

Catalan J, Gath DH, Bond A, Day A, Hall L (1991). Evaluation of a brief psychological treatment for emotional disorders in primary care. *Psychological Medicine* **21**; 1013–1018.

Cooper B, Sylph J (1973). Life events in the onset of neurotic illness: an investigation in general practice. *Psychological Medicine* **3**; 421–435.

Cooper P, Osborn M, Gath D, Feggetter G (1982). Evaluation of a modified self-report measure of social adjustments. *British Journal of Psychiatry* **141**; 68–75.

Croft–Jeffreys JC, Wilkinson G (1989). Estimated cost of neurotic disorders in UK general practice 1985. *Psychological Medicine* **19**; 549–558.

D'Zurilla TJ, Godfried MR (1971). Problem solving and behaviour modification. *Journal of Abnormal Psychology* **78**; 107–126.

DeRubeis RJ, Hollon SD, Grove W, Evans MD, Garvey MJ, Tuason VB (1990). How does cognitive therapy work? Cognitive change and symptom change in cognitive therapy and pharmacotherapy for depression. *Journal of Consulting and Clinical Psychology* **58(6)**; 862–869.

Didjurjeit U, Kruse J, Smitz N, Stuckenschneider P, Sawickip P (2002). A time limited problem orientated psychotherapeutic intervention in type 1 diabetic patients with complications. A randomised control trial. *Diabetic Medicine* **19**; 814–821.

Dowrick C, Dunn G, Ayuso–Mateos JL, Dalgard O, Page H, Lehtinen V, *et al.* (2000). Problem-solving treatment and group psychoeducation for depression: multicentre randomised controlled trial. *British Medical Journal* **321**; 1450–1454.

Evans J, Williams JMG, O'Laughlin S, Howells K (1992). Autobiographical memory in problem-solving strategies of para-suicide patients. *Psychological Medicine* **22**; 399–405.

Evans K, Tyrer P, Catalan J, Schmidt U, Davidson K, Dent J, *et al.* (1999). Manual-assisted cognitive-behaviour therapy 9MACT: a randomized controlled trial of a brief intervention with bibliotherapy in the treatment of recurrent deliberate self-harm. *Psychological Medicine* **29**; 19–25.

Falloon I, *et al.* (1984). Relapse: a reappraisal of assessment of outcome in schizophrenia. *Schizophrenia Bulletin* **10(2)**; 293–299.

Fava M, Bless E, Otto MW, Pava JA, Rosenbaum JF (1994). Dysfunctional attitudes in major depression changes with pharmacotherapy. *The Journal of Nervous and Mental Disease* **182**; 45–49.

Fawcett J, Epstein P, Fiester SJ, Ellan J, Autry J (1987). Clinical management—imipramine/placebo administration manual. *Psychopharmacological Bulletin* **23**; 309–324.

Frank E, Prien RF, Jarrett RB, Keller MB, Kupfer DJ, Lavori PW, *et al.* (1991). Conceptualization and rationale for consenus definitions of terms in major depressive disorder: remission, recovery, relapse and recurrence. *Archives of General Psychiatry* **48**; 851–855.

Geddes J, Butler R (2001). Depressive disorders. *Clinical Evidence* **5**; 652–667.

Gibbons JS, Butler J, Urwin P, Gibbsons JL (1978). Evaluation of a social work service for self-poisoning patients. *British Journal of Psychiatry* **133**; 111–118.

Ginsberg G, Marks I, Walters H (1984). Cost benefit analysis of a controlled trial of nurse therapy for neurosis in primary care. *Psychological Medicine* **14**; 683–690.

Goldberg D, Huxley P (1992). *Common mental disorders by a social model.* Routledge, London.

Hamilton M (1967). Development of a rating scale for primary depressive illness. *British Journal of Social and Clinical Psychology* **6**; 278–296.

Hawton K, Catalan J (1987). *Attempted Suicide: A Practical Guide to its Nature and Management*, 2nd edn, Oxford University Press: Oxford.

Hawton K, McKeown S, Day A, Martin P, O'Connor M, Yule J (1987). Evaluation of out-patient counselling compared with general practitioner care following overdoses. *Psychological Medicine* **17**; 751–761.

Hawton K, Kirk J (1989). Problem-solving. In: *Cognitive behaviour therapy for psychiatric problems* (eds. Hawton K, Salkovskis P, Kirk J, Clark D). Oxford University Press, Oxford, pp. 406–426.

Houts PS, Nezu AM, Nezu CM, Boucher JA (1996). The prepared family care giver. A problem-solving approach to family care giver education. *Patient Education and Counselling* **27**; 63–73.

Jenkins R, Lewis G, Bebbington P, Brugha T, Farrell M, Gill B, *et al.* (1997). The National Psychiatric Morbidity Surveys of Great Britain—initial findings from the Household Survey. *Psychological Medicine* **27**; 775–778.

Johnson DAW, Mellor M (1977). The severity of depression in patients treated in general practice. *Journal of the Royal College of General Practitioners* **27**; 419–422.

Johnson DAW (1981). Depression: treatment compliance in general practice. *Acta Psychiatria Scandinavia* **291** (suppl.); 447–463.

Katon W, Von Korff M, Lin E, Walker E, Simon G, Bush T, *et al.* (1995). A collaborative management to achieve treatment guidelines impact on depression in primary care. *JAMA* **273**; 1026–31.

Katon W, Robinson P, Von Korff M, Lin E, Bush T, Ludman E, *et al.* (1996). A multi-faceted intervention to improve treatment of depression in primary care. *Archives of General Psychiatry* **53**; 924–32.

Katon W, Von Korff M, Lin E, Simon G, Walker E, Unutzer J, *et al.* (1999). Stepped collaborative care for primary care patients with persistent symptoms of depression. A randomised trial. *Archives of General Psychiatry* **56**; 1109–15.

Lewinsohn PM, Libet J (1972). Pleasant events activity schedules and depression. *Journal of Abnormal Psychology* **79**, 291–295.

Liepman R, Covey L, Shapiro A (1979). The Hopkins symptom checklist. *Journal of Affective Disorders* **1**; 9–24.

Linehan MM, Camper P, Chiles JA, Strohsahl K, Shearin EN (1987). Interpersonal problem solving and parasuicide. *Cognitive Therapy and Research* **11**, 1–12.

Lloyd KR, Jenkins R, Mann A (1996). Long term outcome of patients with neurotic disorder in general practice. *British Medical Journal* **313**; 26–28.

McCormick A, Fleming D, Charton J, OPCS (1995). *Morbidity statistics in general practice: fourth national study, 1991–1992.* HMSO, London.

McLeavy BC, Daly RJ, Ludgate JW, Murray CM (1994). Interpersonal problem-solving skill training in the treatment of self-poisoning patients. *Suicide and Life-Threatening Behavior* **24**, 382–394.

Mann AH, Jenkins R, Belsey E (1981). The 12 month outcome of patients with neurotic illness in general practice. *Psychological Medicine* **11**; 535–50.

Mulhall DJ (1976). Systematic self-assessment by PQRST (Personal Questionnaire Rapid Scaling Technique). *Psychological Medicine* **5**; 591–597.

Murray CJ, Lopez AD (1996). *The global burden of disease: a comprehensive assessment of mortality and disability from disease, injuries and risk factors in 1990 and projected to 2020*. Boston Mass., Harvard School of Public Health on behalf of the World Health Organisation and the World Bank.

Mynors–Wallis LM, Gath DH, Lloyd–Thomas AR, Tomlinson D (1995). Randomised controlled trial comparing problem-solving treatment with amitriptyline and placebo for major depression in primary care. *British Medical Journal* **310**; 441–445.

Mynors-Wallis L (1996). Problem solving treatment. Evidence for effectiveness and feasibility in Primary Care. *International Journal of Psychiatry and Medicine* **26**; 249–62.

Mynors–Wallis LM, Gath D, Davies I, Gray A, Barbour F (1997). A randomised controlled trial and cost analysis of problem-solving treatment given by community nurses for emotional disorders in primary care. *British Journal of Psychiatry* **170**; 113–119.

Mynors–Wallis LM, Gath D, Day A, Baker F (2000). Randomised controlled trial of problem-solving treatment, antidepressant medication and combined treatment for major depression in primary care. *British Medical Journal* **320**; 26–30.

Mynors-Wallis L (2002). Does problem solving treatment work through resolving problems. *Psychological Medicine* **32**; 1315–19.

National Institute for Clinical Excellence (2004). *Management of depression in primary and secondary care—Clinical Guideline 23.*

Nezu A (1986). Efficacy of a social problem-solving therapy approach for unipolar depression. *Journal of Consulting and Clinical Psychology* **54**; 196–202.

Nezu AM, Nezu CM, Perri MG (1989). *Problem-solving therapy for depression.* Wiley, New York.

Patsiokas AT, Clum GA (1985). Effects of psychotherapeutic strategies in the treatment of suicide. *Psychotherapy* **22**, 281–290.

Paykel ES, Hart D, Priest RG (1998). Changes in public attitudes to depression during the Defeat Depression Campaign. *British Journal of Psychiatry* **173**; 519–22.

Perri MG, Nezu AM, McKelvey WF, Shermer RL, Renjilian DA, Viegener BJ (2001). Relapse prevention training and problem-solving therapy in the long term management of obesity. *Journal of Consulting and Clinical Psychology* **69**; 722–726.

Salkovskis PM, Ather AC, Storer D (1990). Cognitive behavioural problem-solving in the treatment of patients who repeatedly attempt suicide. *British Journal of Psychiatry* **157**; 871–876.

Schotte DE, Clum GA (1987). Problem-solving skills in psychiatric patients. *Journal of Consulting and Clinical Psychology* **55**, 49–54.

Schwartz MD, Lurman C, Audrain J, Cella D, River B, Stefanek M, *et al.* (1998). The impact of brief problem-solving training intervention for relatives of recently diagnosed breast cancer patients. *Anals of Behavioural Medicine* **20**; 7–12.

Scott J (1998). Psychological treatments for depression. In: *Clinical topics in psychotherapy* (ed. Digby C). Royal College of Psychiatrists, London.

Simons AD, Garfield SL, Murphy GE (1984). The process of change in cognitive therapy and pharmacotherapy for depression. *Archives of General Psychiatry* **41**; 45–51.

Simons L, Mynors–Wallis LM, Pickering R, Gray A, Brooking J, Thompson C, *et al.* (2001). A randomised controlled trial of problem-solving for anxiety, depression and life difficulties by community psychiatric nurses among general practice patients: background and method. *Primary Care Psychiatry* **7(4)**; 129–135.

Thomas CM, Morris S (2003). Cost of depression among adults in England in 2000. *British Journal of Psychiatry* **183**; 514–19.

Townsend E, Hawton K, Alterman DG, Arensman E, Gunnell D, Hazell P, *et al.* (2001). The efficacy of problem-solving treatment after deliberate self-harm; meta-analysis of randomised control trials with respect to depression, hopelessness and improvement in problems. *Psychological Medicine* **31(6)**; 979–988.

Unutzer J, Rubenstein L, Caton W, Tang L, Duan N, Wells KB (2003). Two effects of quality improvement programmes on medication and management for depression. *Archives of General Psychiatry* **58**; 934–42.

Wells KB, Stewart A, Hays RD, Burnam MA, Rogers W, Daniels M, *et al.* (1989). The functioning and well-being of depressed patients from the Medical Outcomes Study. *Journal of the American Medical Association* **262**; 914–919.

Wilkinson G, Allen P, Marshall G (1993). The role of the practice nurse in the management of depression in general practice: treatment adherence to antidepressant medication. *Psychological Medicine* **23**; 229–239.

Williams J, Barrett J, Oxman T, *et al.* (2000). Treatment of dysthymia and minor depression in primary care: a randomised trial comparing placebo, paroxetine, and problem-solving therapy. *Journal of the American Medical Association* **284**; 1570–1572.

Wing JK, Hooper JE, Sartorius N (1974). *The measurement and classification of psychiatric symptoms*. Cambridge University Press, Cambridge.

Wood B, Mynors–Wallis LM (1997). Problem-solving treatment for patients in palliative care. *Palliative Medicine* **11**; 49–54.

Index

Note to Index: PST = problem-solving treatment